Putting Your Best Feet Forward

A Guide to Feet Care

Kevin Harmon

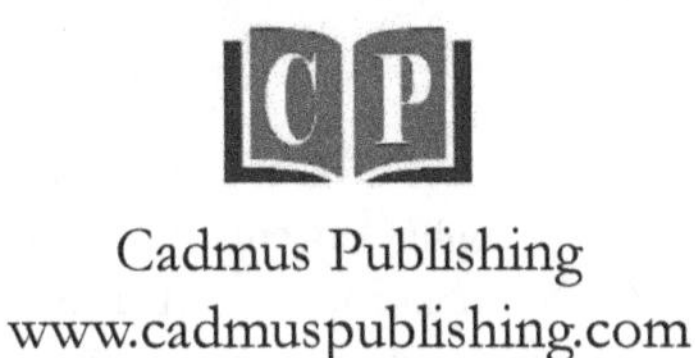

Cadmus Publishing
www.cadmuspublishing.com

TABLE OF CONTENTS

Why a Book About Feet?

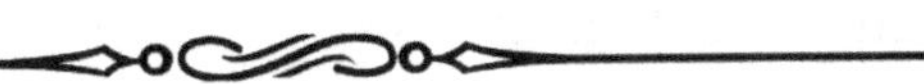

Although I've had issues with my one poor foot for most of my life, the notion of writing a book centering on feet wellness didn't enter my constantly-racing mind until I participated in my first half-marathon in my hometown of Chicago. Not only was I ill-prepared condition-wise to run 13.1 miles for the first time ever, it rained heavily during the entire event, my suffering feet got soaked, tired and blistered to the point that by the time I got home several hours later, I could hardly walk. It was if all the years of issues, abuse and mileage I'd put on my unbalanced feet were hitting me that Sunday morning. If I was in a Flintstones cartoon my feet would have been pulsating like boulders fell on top of them.

My foot issues started at an early age. As a kid, I was playing in our home with a female cousin and while running after her I stepped on a tack that left this deep, painful wound and re-emerging scar that I not only never got medical treatment for, but was something that lingered on for years causing me problems. Additionally, I was born with no arch in my left foot that was also severely flat, not to mention funny-looking. That created an alignment imbalance. To make matters worse, my left leg is slightly shorter by a few centimeters than the right, resulting in me having a distinct gait that I was not only teased about during those formative years, but also caused discomfort in other parts of my body as well. The combination of these things affected my self-esteem and self-image, as well my emotional and physical well-being.

Despite this, I was still able to participate and be pretty good at sports. But as my body grew and I gained weight, the pain in my feet became more of an issue. It was mostly in my left foot but my poor right foot had to compensate so much it suffered in discomfort too. Because of a problematic and chaotic childhood, sports, along with writing became my escape from my physical and emotional pain. The misfortune hit again. I was looking forward to my senior year of high school basketball in Chicago's Public League, setting myself up to get a scholarship at a high-level university. During the first game of the season, with my brother and girlfriend in the crowd cheering me on, I suffered a severe stress fracture in the supposedly normal right foot.

It was near the end of the first quarter, someone from my team had missed a jump shot and I tried retrieving the basketball headed for the corner of the court, eventually got to it and tried turning and shooting in the same motion before the buzzer went off ending the quarter. I felt something pop, but tried to keep playing knowing that some college recruiters were in the stands. For a left-handed player like me, we push off our right foot for power, stability and explosion and with this injury I couldn't push at all. For some reason, I never saw a doctor, I figured this was something that would heal on it's own fairly quickly. It didn't.

I kept trying to rush back into the lineup but the pain was too unbearable. I missed most of my senior year, lost conditioning and this pretty much killed my chances of playing college basketball on a higher level. I neglected my feet care. I did end up playing at a small college in Wisconsin.

During my freshman year, all the pre-season conditioning took its toll on me. The injury had not healed one hundred percent, my body began compensating, resulting in an altered posture, then severe lower back pain. We had trainers and I was always getting treatment for my feet and back. Nike was the shoe company our school had a contract with, but Nike basketball shoes back in the 1980s didn't jive with my narrow feet and ankles. Plus, I was lifting weights for the first time and was on a pretty good nutrition plan, a benefit of being a scholarship athlete. I gained weight and muscle, going from 165 pounds to 190 in a year. That added weight did help me on the basketball court, being able to take bumps and pushes while driving to the basket, but this simultaneously resulted in more pain for my lower back and feet. My upper body was denser, more muscular adding more pressure on my back and feet.

For some reason the problems leveled off for most of my 20s and 30s, even though I was still playing a lot of recreational basketball, softball, cycling, running, skiing and climbing. I became so passionate about fitness, body mechanics and nutrition, eventually transitioning from life as a newspaper sports reporter to a personal fitness trainer and personal chef after going back to school to obtain degrees in health education and culinary arts.

Age brought about more acute feet issues. I noticed my balance being off - this was exposed when I seriously got into yoga, which lets you know pretty quickly when one side of your body is stronger than the other and your body is out of alignment. I started wearing orthodic inserts in my shoes and made it my business to learn all I could about feet, balance and posture wellness so that I wouldn't be a messed up person in my older years. I can't tell you how many people I've seen walking around with seemingly feet-related issues.

I was fortunate enough to get a freelance assignment to do a fitness story for a magazine focusing on preventative feet care for workers in the hospitality industry - nail technicians, massage therapists, restaurant servers, hotel workers, etc. During my research, I learned a lot. The magazine's editor suggested I flush out my findings a bit more and make a book out of it. Hey, it sounded like a good idea for me to tackle - why keep all this juicy knowledge to myself?

So this book - *Putting Your Best Foot Forward* - is all about the science and care of feet, including balance and posture treatments, which are all connected. I can thank a spa technician at the Copper Mountain Ski Resort in Summit County, Colorado for opening my eyes to natural treatments for the feet, hands and face. I gotta be honest, I initially thought all the claims made by tecnicians while getting those spa treatments were bogus and just a way to get people to spend a lot of money while at the resorts. I couldn't have been more wrong and I'm reminded that education is the key to eliminating ignorant and ill-informed perceptions of most situations.

Additionally, any wellness book would be incomplete without addressing the importance of feet care. Recent science indicated three of four people experience, or have experienced feet pain in their life. Feet issues can lead to a myriad of problems, creating imbalances elsewhere in your body while generally making your life miserable. I've spent many hours and lots of money paying for massage, reflexology, acupuncture, naprapathy, pediatric and physical therapy treatments over the years. Fortunately, I've gotten enough professional help to maintain an active and mostly pain-free life.

Ever notice how folks with feet pain often ironically have back pain too? That was me. I've also had knee pain as well as I've gotten older, especially when I walk longer distances. It's sad to say, but even as a fitness professional, I was ignorant to some of the bio-mechanic connections between feet and body.

I've also started stretching and doing more yoga, something that didn't happen until I got in my 50s. Expanding my yoga practice to include more feet and balance work, combined with targeting my resistance training to include more functional fitness training, has proved more beneficial too.

I eat well probably seventy-five percent of the time and have kept my weight in check, consuming more power foods as I age. This is my passion and I know people struggling in this area and I try to provide tiny things here and there as a personal fitness trainer and personal chef to help. Feet problems might not life threatening, but they can be lifestyle altering. Like I mentioned earlier, feet pain can be the triggering event to musculoskeletal problems resulting in a loss of mobility.

In 2022, about twenty-four percent over the age of 45 suffered from feet pain, according to a study I read. For someone over seventy, it's more like fifty percent. Until I started researching and talking to people for this project, I just figured feet pain was a normal part of aging. I remember being on a bus and judging the folks who would get on the bus, then off after a few blocks, thinking judgmentally they were too lazy to walk such a short distance. Now I see this differently as I studied more clearly that some of these folks moved as if they were indeed in pain. Some were overweight, some not. I did notice gait and balance issues too.

I've written quite a few articles for fitness publications and going back to school helped me to understand stuff like plantar fasciitis, heel spurs, bunions, corns and arthritic-related stuff. I've lived many of these issues. It's not cool to have unhappy feet. Vascular, nerve, skin and issues related to weight gain or diabetes are real and serious stuff that everyday people deal with.

My skin issues started when I was a kid. I was ten when I noticed breakout, all over the place and dry skin on my elbows and feet. Looking back on those days knowing what I know now, the skin issues started right around the same time the sexual abuse I suffered started for the first time. There were other traumatic and chaotic events in my life going on, such as my mom's mental breakdown and subsequent institutionalization in a mental health facility.

I had a very stressful and depressing childhood on many levels. My biological dad left us when I was very young, then my mom re-married an alcoholic. I was such a lonely and lost kid, battling bullies, loneliness, depression and anxiety. It was strange to me that these skin problems seems to come and go. When the symptoms were really bad, I would notice breakouts all around my face, around my eyebrows, under my chin. When I was thirteen and started growing a mustache I had dry skin and breakouts around it. Playing sports and having to answer questions about my skin because a source of stress and embarrassment for me. Trying to cope with my mom's mental illness and now my struggles was a lot to deal with.

There were other things going on that were indicators I was under a lot of stress. Hiccups. Athlete's Feet, also called Tinea Pedis. This is a fungus. An itchy gray, white or red rash that shows up on the bottoms of the feet and in between the toes. All these things were problematic all through high school and college. I would get such severe breakouts on my hands I would go through what it seemed like a bottle of lotion or a container of medicated cream every week or so. I actually tried all kinds of lotions, creams, ointments - nothing worked. I thought I had haunted feet!

Years after I started doing some research and finally deciding to ask a doctor about my condition, I found out I had eczema. What the hell is eczema anyway?, I wondered.

The doctor said it was a long-term, autoimmune skin condition that can come and go for years and family history can be one cause of it, stress another. I unfortunately checked both of those boxes. My mom had eczema, my son Taylor did too when he was little. Stress has ignited eczema for most of my life. The stress of childhood abuse and trauma, being a high level high school and college athlete, a journalist reporting for newspapers, the ups and downs of relationships combined with my own addictions have played a role in eczema breakouts over the years.

I read all I could about eczema and even tried an eczema diet for a while, cutting out processed, highly acidic foods and most sugars and salts from my diet. Eczema can be a big deal like other inflammatory skin conditions such as psoriasis, rosacea and dermatitis. I tried hard dealing with my eczema once I figured out that was what I had. There were two main types that I did lots of research on, two types of eczema I thought were applicable for me - asteatotic eczema and pompholyx eczema. Asteatotic happens as the result of aging, nutritional deficiencies and can be triggered by irritants likes certain soaps and detergents. Pompholyx is ignited by stress (me) and some environmental triggers. Both can be activated also by eating lots of inflammatory stuff such as processed and highly acidic foods like deli meats, sausages and sugars.

I initially tried using foods and supplements loaded with powers supposedly great for those suffering skin issues - vitamin B-6, biotin, magnesium, vitamin-C, zinc, Omega-3, vitamin-D, calcium. Family history and stress were the main reasons for my eczema, an overly acidic condition where your body processes excess acid, which is a part of the inflammation process.

I would also try all sorts of over-the-counter products at Walgreens, CVS, Walmart and other stores. Eventually, I had a long talk with my primary care physician and she referred me to a specialist who prescribed several products that only provided minimal results.

As luck would have it, I started working as a quality control inspector for a health and beauty products contract manufacturing company. We made everything from deodorant, hair and skin care products, Epsom salts and more. One of my goals while working there was to learn as much as I could about the products and the solutions they supposedly provided for those of us with skin issues.

I learned so much so fast. I picked the minds of the general manager, the woman who hired me, she had previously worked for a variety of beauty companies in the past and was a wealth of knowledge when it came to the ends and outs of this industry. It was like I was in two worlds there. One, on the production floor I dealt with line workers, line leaders and the production managers. In the office, I kicked it with a cosmetic chemist, some research and development folks, the people who purchased raw materials and my boss, the quality control manager, who overwhelmed me with information.

It was enjoyable and educational learning so much about this industry. I'd been to spas and knew quite a bit about skin care, the power of exfoliation, how the base of a good skin scrub included a moisturizer, exfoliate and antioxidant of some kind, plus a good oil.

Then COVID-19 hit and I had a lot of time on my hands in my apartment, with so much in my community being shut down. I was older and it seemed like my skin issues were more severe when there was a breakout. So I started experimenting with products, trying to come up with my own all-natural solutions to my skin problems.

Like I said, eczema is an overly acidic condition where your body produces excess acid, which is a part of inflammation. It really has no cure and I figured since I may be stuck with it for the rest of my life, I might as well attack it.

I was motivated by an experience with my grandmother. She was living in an assistant living facility and had many issues affecting her dexterity such as arthritis. She was on a lot of medication and I noticed how dehydrated she looked. She didn't have enough strength to paint her nails or even open a bottle of pills. I would try out some of my experimental scrubs and moisturizers on her and I saw huge differences in her aging and medicated skin. My grandmother said I had a gift for healing and I should consider selling my skin healing products commercially. I used my family and some friends as test pilots to see if I had something worth pursuing more.

My grandmother also suffered from eczema. To put it in the simplest terms, with eczema the mortar that holds your skin cells together breaks down because of dryness and that makes your skin prone to inflammation. Because it's exposed from the outside, this looks like dry, red rashes that can be itchy or flaky. It can get especially bad in cold weather months when your skin losses moisture more easily. Moisture is like putting mortar back between bricks. I read books and researched online all I could about eczema.

THE BENEFITS OF YOGA ON YOUR FEET

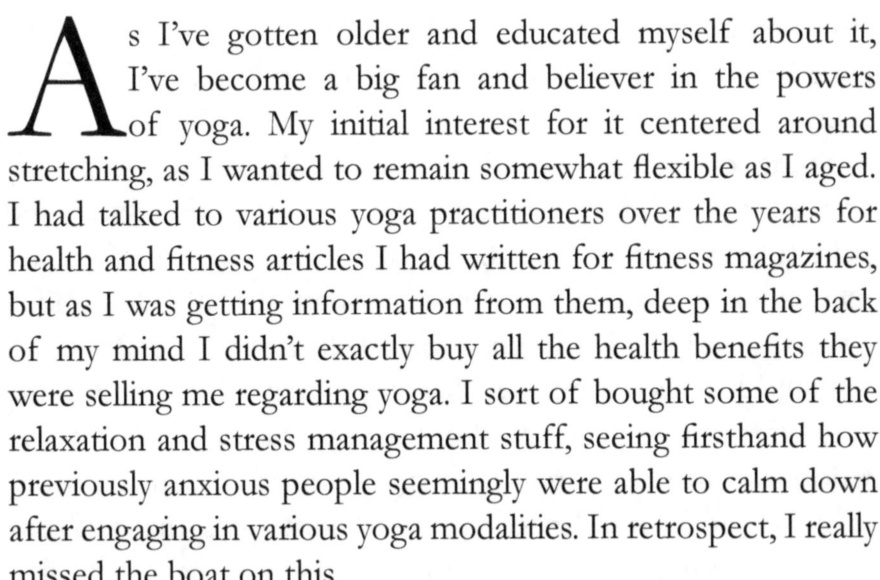

As I've gotten older and educated myself about it, I've become a big fan and believer in the powers of yoga. My initial interest for it centered around stretching, as I wanted to remain somewhat flexible as I aged. I had talked to various yoga practitioners over the years for health and fitness articles I had written for fitness magazines, but as I was getting information from them, deep in the back of my mind I didn't exactly buy all the health benefits they were selling me regarding yoga. I sort of bought some of the relaxation and stress management stuff, seeing firsthand how previously anxious people seemingly were able to calm down after engaging in various yoga modalities. In retrospect, I really missed the boat on this.

Then I met a teacher I was talking to after a yoga class about the back and foot pain I had. She went into this in-depth conversation regarding some bio-mechanic dynamics, about how one part of the body is usually stronger and better adjusted than the other, and that by engaging in a consistent yoga practice you can create balance within your body that could help alleviate pain. Turns out she wasn't just pontificating, she was right. When I first started doing yoga, I could tell as a left-handed person the left side of my body was stronger and more flexible than the right side. Because my left foot is flat and my left leg is a few centimeters shorter than the right, I've struggled with balance and alignment issues over the course of my life. Many of the standing poses I was taught initially helped tremendously with my left foot and lower back pain.

Yoga helped me calm down too. You can't be in a rush doing the different asanas, or poses, or you could hurt yourself. Yoga really is a transformative journey and has long been known as a great antidote for stress and by combining stress-reducing techniques, while teaching you to control your breathing, you can truly clear your mind and relax your body.

Some of the physical benefits include greater flexibility and strength, better muscle tone, balance, breathing and pain tolerance. Some of the mental benefits include greater mental calmness, better stress reduction capability, body awareness, along with generating feelings of serenity. I can say all this has been true for me. I have been practicing various forms of yoga for about five years now. As a person who has suffered through anxiety, depression and various forms of addiction, I needed to find something that not only helped me physically, but spiritually and emotionally as well.

Being a consistent yoga practitioner has resulted in a better overall mood, as well as helping me with my balance, posture and to lengthen my aging spine, a concern for many of us. It's helped strengthen the bones, muscles and ligaments in my feet and ankles too. There are practices that primarily work on these areas. Although they don't show your age like other bodyparts, our feet flatten out and grow as we age. They get stiff and the muscles need to be exercised regularly.

There are so many books, CDs and DVDs out there on the many aspects of yoga, as well as magazines such as *Yoga Journal* and in my neck of the woods, *Yoga Chicago,* that offer instruction. Since this book is about feet wellness, I'll get more specific about its correlation with yoga. With my feet/leg/back issues, at the advice of a fellow personal fitness trainer friend, I initially tried a Iyengar Yoga class, which focused on very precise alignment, deep stretching while holding poses longer. This helped me with some of my imbalances. There was a lot of uni-lateral stuff in this class as well, like standing and bending and stretching on one leg at a time. That motivated me enough to try other Yoga classes including chair yoga, which incorporated many poses for the feet.

All those toe flexes, ankle twisting, calf raises, etc., brought on by yoga helps with blood flow, circulation and inflammation, which is a major cause of feet pain. A lack of activity for your feet is a major reason many folks have feet problems and yoga can be a simple, low-impact way to deal with feet issues. Not everyone can run, walk, cycle, but many of the stationary aspects of yoga can be done safety and effectively.

Many yoga postures also target your hamstrings, back, core, legs and even shoulders, which can all be related to your feet, which serve as a foundation for your body. Doing moves one leg at a time really does help with balance, another consideration that can contribute to feet problems. It takes tons of patience to do this stuff.

Having a strong core helps with many things including your feet. It's our center of gravity and is made up of a set of trunk muscles that serve to stabilize us, helping with posture and balance. I've dive more into core considerations in another chapter.

It can be overwhelming trying to master all of the yoga moves that can be good for your feet, posture and balance, but I thought I would briefly touch on some of my favorites.

1. Yogi toes - To help improve your balance, while standing or seated in a chair, spread your toes as wide as possible and slowly place them firmly down on a flat surface. Repeat this.

2. Ankle pumps - In this move you can either do it sitting in a chair or laying down on the floor. All you will do is go back and forth from pointing your toes like a ballet dancer and then flexing your ankles.

3. Inversion and eversion - Sit in a chair and simply turn the soles of your feet toward each other (inversion) and then turn the soles away from each other (eversion), then repeat. This is a great exercise to warm up those ankles.

4. Squeeze and release - Squeeze your feet muscles by curling your toes and then releasing. Do this up to five times to help your feet relax.

I took a yoga class once and the instructor said, after I was talking to her about some of my feet problems, that I might like to try her toega class. Yes, toega. She said it was a class that focused on some yoga and stretching postures for the toes that could help my balance, foot and heel pain. I enjoyed it and I felt the flexibility in my feet being better and after a few sessions I did notice a difference in my posture and balance.

EMBRACE THE HEALING POWERS OF WATER

The first time I experienced the healing powers of water I was a skinny, freshman college basketball player, who, after a grueling, preseason conditioning session, found myself in a powerful whirlpool bath for injury-related treatment for the first time. My foot was killing me. This was less than a year removed from the stress fracture of my left foot that I suffered in high school and the basketball shoes that the University of Wisconsin at Superior had a contract with, Niké, didn't fit right for my damaged flat foot, as well as narrow ankles.

Fortunately, one of our athletic trainers knew a thing or two about treating feet pain - she was a former college track and cross-country runner and had her fair share of shin, feet and ankle problems. She suggested I try this extremely hot water, whirlpool bath before I did anything else. She provided me a long explanation about the healing power of fast-moving waters and how this helped with circulation and pain relief, among other things.

Flash forward many years later -my wife Dianne and I were at Colorado's Copper Mountain Ski Resort and my feet were and shins were killing me after several hours on the intermediate and advanced slopes. At the resort's spa in the fitness center, one of the spa's technicians overheard me complaining to my wife about how my dogs were killing me in this high altitude wonderland, and she suggested I try this feet soak in a circulating little whirlpool they had that had a mixture of salts and herbs spinning in a clockwise motion. The technician said certain plants and salts have medicinal powers that work in sync with fast-moving waters.

Externally, I was never more shocked at how healthy my skin looked and how shiny my toenails looked after the spa session. It reminded me of visiting my brother when he lived in Hawaii and coming out of the salty and mineral-rich Pacific Ocean waters and when Dianne and I got out of the water it looked like we had the most dynamic feet and hand scrub ever.

I remember someone commenting to us in the elevator at the hotel we were staying after leaving the beach how healthy and rich our feet and toenails looked. I would later find out the fast-moving, mineral-saturated, salty ocean water helped to purify the skin like a deep skin polish while refreshing our feet too. That is what getting this session at Copper Mountain's spa reminded me of.

I say all of this to urge consideration in investing in a good whirlpool-based spa session once in a while, letting the healing motion of moving water treat you. It can improve circulation, relax tight muscles while doing other good things. If getting a spa session is out of your budget, perhaps invest, like I did, in a small portable whirlpool bath. Fill it with hot water and add Epsom salt - the magnesium in it is great for tired and sore feet. You can also get a device that can help the water circulate more. Water can be a great healer in many ways.

I'm a big fan of all types of hydrotherapy and highly recommend in experimenting with them to find the right one that fits for you. Just make sure you have on hand essential oils, exfoliation products, a rough brush and a wash cloth. I speak a lot about essential oils when I write elsewhere in this book about aromatherapy. For a perfect healing water treatment I would use about five drops of essential oil in the moving waters. Almond and avocado oils are great for bunions and inflamed joints. Grapefruit and tea tree oil works well for corns, calluses and Athlete's Feet.

My favorite feet treatment

Three tablespoons oatmeal
one-fourth cup tea tree oil
one teaspoon baking soda
two tablespoons salt
After soaking feet in a foot basin or whirlpool tub, mix oats in a Magic Bullet or small blender, then put in bowl and mix with other ingredients with a spoon, rub on feet to exfoliate, then wash off.

A soothing feet treatment

Five drops essential oil (like thyme or rosemary)
one cup apple cider vinegar
one cup Epsom salt

Drop all ingredients in a hydro feet basin and soak feet. This treatment can provide relief for inflamed joints, Athlete's Feet and arch pain. The water should be between 95-116 degrees.

Wine-based feet treatment

One bottle of medium-bodied red wine, such as Pinot Noir
one cup Epsom salt
one cup olive oil
Pull all ingredients in a hydro feet basin, or large bucket and soak feet for at least 20 minutes. The wine provides a nice antioxidant for the skin, the oil moisturizes the skin and the Epsom salt can soothe aching feet.

Another name for the healing powers of water is aqua therapy. I've used this when training clients that I worked with as a fitness trainer at several hospital-based fitness centers that had a pool or whirlpool on hand. I initially tried aqua therapy in college when trying to rehabilitate from injuries while also dealing with my longstanding foot issues.

Aqua therapy is great for seniors and any aging body, really. There are a lot of exercises geared towards the feet. It works at supplying energy, targeting flexibility while also providing cardiovascular flexibility to the body. For example. A hydro splash aquatic class uses buoys, noodles, weights and other suspended-in-water techniques to stretch muscles, focusing often on the core while also helping gain more strength and flexibility. The suspended-in-water aspect takes folks off their feet, which provides less impact and stress on the joints by decreasing weight bearing activities. It can help tone muscles, increase flexibility and balance.

It's easier to move around in water. I've taken many aqua therapy classes and find them a great supplement to the resistance, cardiovascular and balance training I was already doing. It's also a great introduction for someone who hasn't done any resistance work, or for someone simply just interested in functional fitness.

Working at hospital-based fitness centers, which often specializes in rehabilitative work, I found aqua therapy in particular, and the healing powers of water in general, were used quite a bit to help previously inactive people move more towards a low-impact fitness program. It was effective for me as I used aqua therapy almost exclusively when I was recovering from a skiing accident.

More about water

Any feet health book would be incomplete without something being said about the consumption of water. Water is good for just about everything in your body, including your feet. It's good for your skin and for normal bodily functioning. Water is in every cell of your body and most people would be surprised to know that your feet can suffer from you not drinking enough water in the day.

Your body is made up of about sixty percent water, body fat is about ten percent water, your brain is about eighty-five percent water, your muscles contain about seventy-five percent water, your bones about twenty-two percent water and your blood contains about seventy percent water. Every organ and tissue in your body contains water.

Your body needs water to maintain body temperature and uses water to get rid of waste products through perspiration, urination and bowel movements. Water cushions and lubricates the joints and protects the spinal cord. It carries nutrients to the cells and helps you digest your food. Water is needed to absorb certain hormones and gives muscles their natural ability to contract and maintain muscle tone. Water is extremely important for maintaining great skin - it helps prevent sagging skin that follows extreme weight loss, and it softens the skin and reduces wrinkles. Hydrated feet helps ward off many potential problems.

Although you get about eighty percent of the water you need from the drinks you consume during the day, the remaining twenty percent comes from the food that you eat. Plain water is the best way to hydrate your body. You need to drink more water if you exercise often. You may have heard that you should drink eight glasses of water a day and that might not be true depending on your weight and the amount of physical activity that you get. It depends on other factors, like your age and environment. To stay hydrated, you need to drink enough water to replace the water that you lost. Besides losing water everyday through respiration, perspiration, urination and defecation, you lose water in hot weather and humidity, when you have a fever or when you physically exert yourself working or exercising. Your feet lose a lot of water through exercise.

You need to consume enough water to make your urine pale yellow or clear - this is the easiest way to know if you are drinking enough water. If you wait until you are thirsty, your body is most likely dehydrated. When exercising or participating in sports, you should drink eight ounces of water beforehand, four ounces every fifteen minutes during and sixteen ounces of water after your workout. If it's hot and humid, or if you sweat more, you'll need more water.

Remember to stay clear of caffeinated drinks, they dehydrate, not hydrate your body. Here are some other tips to help you hydrate your body.

1. Keep a water bottle with you at all times.
2. Select water over soda, tea or juice when eating out.
3. Drink water before each meal.
4. Drink water from a straw.

If you pee a lot, clear urine is a good indicator that you're getting enough water, but if it's dark and has a bad odor, you need water immediately. Most men need between 80-96 ounces of fluid per day and three liters is about 99 ounces. I try to get one gallon of fluid a day on the days I exercise.

Beware of issues with aging feet

Sometimes when I get up first thing in the morning, then other times when I'm going for a walk, I'm reminded that now I'm an older dude and that I've put a whole bunch of miles on my feet.

It takes me a while whenever I start any exercise movement for my feet to wake up. As much as I hate admitting it, I can't do the same things with my aging feet as I could twenty years ago. When I play basketball, my cuts to the basket are slower and less pronounced, less dramatic. When I jump, the lift off the balls of the balls of my high isn't nearly as high.

I don't run the court nearly as fast and my lateral movement is slower as well. When I ski or snowboard, my carving and twists in the snow are not as crisp as they once were. I can speak from experience that not taking into account your aging feet into your active life can result in injury and other issues.

When I started working at a health and beauty manufacturing factory in my mid-50s, my aging feet didn't take to my new job right away. I jumped right into it, had swelling so bad after the first few weeks that when I got home I had to soak and elevate my feet in an effort to relieve myself of extreme discomfort. I didn't have the right shoes for the job, I should have bought a new pair to deal with walking eight to nine hours constantly on a concrete floor as a quality control inspector. For a person like me with one flat, no-arched foot, this was no joke. I had to take little breaks throughout the course of the night when the pain became unbearable. Just because I considered myself in great shape for my age, I shouldn't have considered myself invincible.

I was involved in sports from the time I started playing Little League baseball until recently - I'm approaching 60 -but still have passion for and engage in all kinds of fitness activities from walking, yoga, circuit training, cycling, weight training, etc. I've learned to have compassion for all the miles and wear and tear I've forced on my feet and have also become mindful not to put the same types of pressure on them than I did even ten years ago.

Seeing a podiatrist regularly is a must, as well as making sure you have the right shoes for a particular activity and a variety of shoes as well, in addition to inserts and insoles if you are engaging in consistent exercise. There are so many muscles in your feet that get worked in a variety of ways depending on what you do that any help your feet will appreciate.

Stretching is also great for aging feet and shouldn't be take lightly and should be done on a regular basis. Stretching doesn't have to be complicated either as there are many simple movements you can do to stretch your feet.

There are injuries that can come as a result of aging feet. Patellofemoral Syndrome, also called runner's knee, is generalized knee pain that can come from years and years of running on hard and uneven surfaces and that knee pain can trickle down to your feet. Plantar fasciitis, an inflammation of the plantar fascia, a web of tough, connective tissue sitting on the bottom of the feet, can also be activated by aging feet moving about on hard and uneven surfaces consistently, inadequate shoes and overuse. Tendinitis, inflammation of a tendon, and bursitis, inflammation of the fluid-filled cushioning sacs between the tendons and the bones, are also injuries that can come from having aging and worn out feet.

Osteoarthritis, caused by worn joint cartilage thereby exposing the joint to surface swelling and edema (fluid buildup), and rheumatoid arthritis, an autoimmune disorder in which the body's immune system attacks joint tissues, are two other common issues that can at least be partially attributed to aging feet. I've also known people who've been active running and walking for a long time to get shin splints, pain felt in the anterior portion of the lower leg that can be caused my muscle imbalances.

Just because you have aging feet doesn't mean you need to give up a life of fitness. It does mean, however, being mindful of what you are doing and how you are doing it, and taking protective measures to ensure you won't have to stop completely at some point.

There has been a lot of debate over supplements, which ones to take and if they are good for you or not. When it comes to aging feet and fighting off inflammation, I suggest giving the following supplements a try. Vitamin D. It's needed for strong bones and overall immunity and it's hard to get it from food alone. Iron. This helps red blood cells carry oxygen throughout your body and women, particularly older women, need more of this than men. If you constantly have cold and tired feet, you may need iron, but have your levels checked with your doctor first.

Calcium works well with vitamin D to help maintain strong bones. Although it might be better to try and get your calcium from food first, the added protection for bones can't hurt as long as you are taking the right amount. I've seen people who've had broken bones in the feet that seemingly took forever to heal.

Collagen. A great protein supplement that's also good for ligaments and tendons. Tendons, made up of fibrous tissue and connects muscles to bone, become more susceptible to injury as we age. Also great for skin and nails if taken consistently.

Omega-3. Found in fish, this supplement is great for among other things, inflammation, which is a common cause of many issues with aging feet.

Magnesium is also good for bone health, zinc, like vitamin D helps with overall metabolism and with wound healing.

INFLAMMATION AND FEET HEALTH

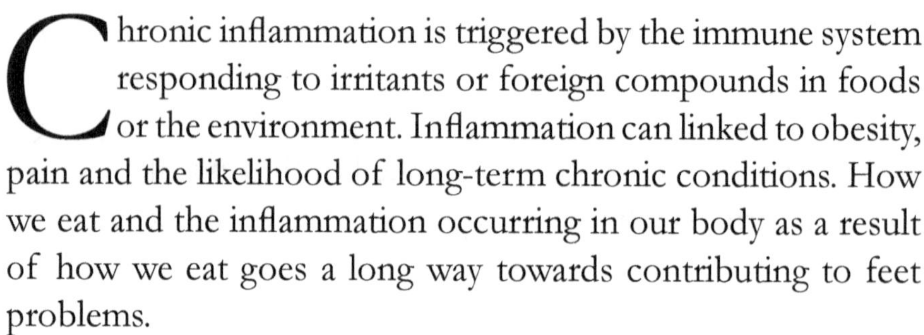

Chronic inflammation is triggered by the immune system responding to irritants or foreign compounds in foods or the environment. Inflammation can linked to obesity, pain and the likelihood of long-term chronic conditions. How we eat and the inflammation occurring in our body as a result of how we eat goes a long way towards contributing to feet problems.

Inflammation can be the cause of feet and ankle pain, swelling and a host of other problems. Look at all the negative salt does to us. We also accelerate inflammation by consuming too many processed foods, sugar, fat and the overall amount of food we consume. We typically eat more than we need and this creates structural concerns that can also cause of host of other issues. As Americans, we typically eat less whole foods than we should, not having enough fruits, vegetables and whole grains in our diet.

The top ten inflammatory subjects are : excessive alcohol, eating too many calories, trans fats, fried foods, refined carbohydrates, too much added sugar including artificial sweeteners, too much salt and not getting enough water.

The key is avoiding inflammation-igniting feet issues and consume as many anti-inflammatory foods as possible. The list of those foods is long. Some of my favorites include cherries, salmon, broccoli, mushrooms, olive oil, avocado, tomatoes, turmeric, spinach/greens, strawberries, citrus fruits, peppers, nuts, cinnamon, vinegar, cucumbers, eggs, Kefir and other probiotic foods and fish. Foods with a high water content helps flush some bad stuff out of your feet and also helps with circulation.

Drinking alkaline water helps too. What you eat affects your urine and other bodily fluids and too much acid in the body, as the result of consuming too many processed foods, can make you more acidic and then your body starts pulling calcium and other minerals to alkaline the body. Our bodies should roughly be eighty percent alkaline and twenty percent acidic. By adding lemon or lime to our water we can change the alkaline and molecular structure to water. Other benefits of consuming more alkaline water include it helping our immune system, aiding in weight loss, energy, skin appearance, digestion, while also controlling inflammation and helping clear toxins from the body.

The absence of inflammation can also result in less feet and ankle pain. Many of us are carrying around too much weight and not eating as well or exercising as much as we should. What speeds up inflammation? A slow metabolism, poor diet, a lack of movement, stress. What slows it down? Fruits, vegetables, lean proteins, exercise, hydration and weight loss.

The more I've learned about inflammation, it makes sense to me how it's linked to nearly every critical disease associated with aging. Although this book focuses on feet care, inflammation is really connected to your whole body. Think about when you have the flu and your body temperature rises to fight the virus - that's a form of inflammation. The same goes with the swelling you get when you sprain an ankle.

Inflammation of the feet can cause various forms of arthritis, lupus and other issues. Although we can't do anything about aging, which increases the chances of inflammation, we can do something about our lifestyle.

I'll elaborate more about the powers of exercise on the feet in other chapters of this book because the fact is the less exercise you get the more likely you are to have some form of inflammation in your body. I did some research and found that around twenty-one percent of people in the United States aged 65-older engaged in regular exercise. That's a good thing.

Feet problems seem more extreme when we're older. From my perspective, the majority of adults become less physically active with age, increasing their risk of developing inflammation and some chronic disease.

Besides inflammation, other physical considerations that come from not exercising: decrease in bone and muscle mass (sarcopenia), decreased balance and coordination, increase in obesity, having a higher percentage of fat mass and osteoarthritis and orthopedic injuries.

THE ROLE OF ANTIOXIDANTS IN NAIL HEALTH

Some of the most powerful weapons you have against aging, tired and rough looking and feeling feet and toes are antioxidants, certain vitamins, minerals and enzymes that take on free radicals that combat the extensive harm they cause to the body. Some common and powerful antioxidants include vitamins A, C, E, B-6 and B-12, along with beta carotene and folic acid. The minerals zinc, selenium and calcium are important too.

I can speak firsthand how consistently consuming antioxidants through foods and supplements has helped with my aging skin, my fight against eczema, Athlete's Feet and providing me better overall energy.

As your body metabolizes food through a process known as oxidation, it also produces nasty by-products called free radicals, which are unstable molecules that can cause significant damage to the body's tissues and contribute to aging of the skin and other biological stuff.

This is where food comes in. One thing to remember is food and antioxidants dance best as a team, so consuming a wide variety by eating many different colored fruits and vegetables is key to getting the most benefits from antioxidants.

The numbers vary on this, but I would say strive to eating about nine servings of fruits and vegetables daily, or to broaden it out between five to thirteen servings daily combined, according to the number of calories consumed. A easy way to attack this would be by trying to have a salad daily, with lots of fruits and vegetables as toppings.

Foods high in biotin like eggs, dairy, cauliflower and greens also are loaded with calcium that's also good for nail health. Again, good nail health can equal good overall feet health. Nuts and seeds help too- they are high in vitamin E and selenium, another powerful trace mineral. Nuts and seeds are great for your metabolism and although a bit calorie-dense, help you stay regular.

Antioxidants also help deal with stress in the body, another cause for weak hair, damaged skin and nails. They are typically low in fat, so you can eat a lot of them. Try to get your antioxidant fruits and vegetables from different colors to avoid getting bored. Not only do antioxidants help with nail health, they can help the feet recover from other things like dry skin and inflammation in the body.

SIMPLE STEPS TO HAPPY FEET

I've had family and friends who've confessed to not being fans of reading an entire book ask me to summarize some simple steps to having happy feet in a concise, one-page narrative. Of course, my first response was "read the whole damn book!"

Eventually I decided to give in. The following steps have come from consulting with several podiatrists that have treated me over the years or served as reference sources for other writing projects.

1. Go barefoot in your home as much as possible. It's good for your feet and helps them breathe.

2. Wear appropriate shoes. Nothing ruins feet more than walking around in shoes that are too small, narrow, etc. For those who care about what others think about your feet/shoes being too big - check your ego and get over it.

3. Don't wear the same shoes everyday. You could be worsening a bad situation with shoes that are worn out or too small. Have several pair in your arsenal.

4. Stay with short heels, your feet will thank you. Heels are feet killers over the long haul.

5. Measure your feet each time you buy shoes. Your feet can grow with age, weight gain, etc.

6. Choose socks that keep sweat away from your feet.

7. Dry your feet throughly coming out of the shower, especially between your toes.

8. Cut your toenails straight across to avoid issues like painful ingrown toenails.

9. Buy your shoes in the evening - that's when your feet are their biggest. Again, don't let your ego be your guide when buying shoes. Comfort and safety is more important than style.

10. Be mindful that your feet swell during exercise so make sure you have the proper shoes and socks on.

11. Remember you should have one finger-width of space between the longest toe to the end of your shoe. Again, a big part of feet issues for some is wearing shoes that are too small and my from my experience from working at a specialty shoe store and being a personal fitness trainer is that women tend to do this more than men. Not being sexist, but it seems women will cram their feet in shoes too small.

12. You need to consistently exercise your feet. The constant circulation helps with overall metabolism. There are all kinds of simple, stationary exercises you can do. Exercising your feet can help improve you overall strength and balance.

As a person who's suffered from unhappy feet for most of his life, I know it's the little steps that need to be taken on a consistent basis to ensure your feet take care of you, especially if you plan to be active for as long as you can. As a fitness guy, it's always perplexed me that people would spend so much time and effort on other parts of their body and neglect their feet. My serious feet care didn't start until I was in my 50s and discovered I had arthritis in one of them.

MORE QUICK HIT SOLUTIONS TO HELP WITH FEET ISSUES

For some reason, some folks think feet care is much more or at least as complicated as addressing other parts of the body that may be problematic, such as the back or shoulders.

The reality is there are many fast options you can address that can prove to be helpful to your feet if you don't wait too long. The following is a list of some solutions.

1. Try to lose some weight, the less pressure on your feet the better. You lose weight quicker through diet than exercise.

2. Eat foods that warm you up, this is called the thermogenic effect - which can help raise metabolism, speed up digestion while helping to to burn calories. Foods such as bananas, ginger, green tea, peanuts and peppers can help. Also, consider a flushing out cleanse of one cup of lemon juice, six cups of water and one teaspoon of salt and have that once a week or so.

3. Consume foods that feed your stomach and keep you full, such as greens, mushrooms, walnuts, oats, black beans, sweet potatoes, eggs, avocado, salmon and the fermented drink Kefir.

4. Consider taking supplements that aid in cardiovascular support for veins, heavy legs, feet and ankles. Omega -3, vitamins B-6, B-12, as well as zinc, magnesium and CoQ-10- an energy supplement. As far as circulation goes, blood goes down the the body and needs support to come back up. If there is no support, that's a recipe for pain, swelling and a buildup of fluids in the legs and feet.

5. Address issues like corns and calluses right away - if they linger they could get worse.

6. Get massage or reflexology sessions to help with pain and other concerns. Educate yourself on self-massage.

7. Try to see a podiatrist as soon as possible and at least yearly to address any concerns.

8. Walk around your house barefoot to help loosen muscles, tendons and ligaments.

Back pain equals feet pain

Back pain can be caused by injury, poor posture, repetitive motion, unhealthy hips or simply by aging. I spent many years of playing basketball outside on concrete courts and I figure that was the cause of some of my back discomfort once I reached my 50s. Our entire body can compensate for back pain and that includes the feet, which takes the brunt of so much punishment.

We can change our gait because of a variety of reasons, and our walking pattern resulting in our feet getting wear in a different way. The soft disks between vertebrae dry over time and those less-subtle disks can be more susceptible to bulging or rupturing and putting pressure on nerves. Conversely, when your spine and pelvis are aligned and your muscles more relaxed, you can be more resilient.

It's difficult to be an active person when the pain in your back affects your feet and how you walk, run, play basketball or even participate in yoga. Fortunately, there are so many fitness things you can do to relieve that back pain to help you do among other things, walk better. You can start by incorporating a variety of yoga poses. Yoga really helped me with my back pain and also to be able to walk with more balance. I started doing yoga in my early 50s with the urging of a friend and got to see how much of a balance difference there was from one side of my body the other.

Some of my favorite yoga poses for back relief are cat and cow, downward dog, locust, bridge, cobra, upward facing dog and plank twists. These moves not only helped with my posture but took so much pressure off my spine. Lifting weights I've spent a lot of time squatting, putting hundreds or pounds of pressure on my back and spine. With my alignment issues it was only a matter of time before problems came. These and other yoga poses have not only helped minimalize my back pain, but helped some of the pain in my left foot be more manageable.

You can also try an exercise ball and by lying on it do all sorts of pelvic isolation and lumbar extensions. Having a medicine ball and doing core exercises can be useful as well. Pilates also wonders for the back.

Speaking of the core, I've had to emphasize many times to my personal training clients that back work isn't complete without doing some core work. Many wanting to work their back ignore their core for some reason. A lot of the strength in our body comes from the core. Thing of your core as a box. You have a front, side and rear portion. Core training, I've learned over the years, is a lot more than just doing crunches.

Think of your back as forming a straight line to your feet. I've see people with back issues lean to one side and others wearing their shoes unevenly, resulting in getting calluses on one side. I've seen others lean forward when they walk because of a weak core, putting pressure on the tops of their feet.

You can also tackle back pain by improving the strength of your hips. I noticed a lot of my back pain went away when I started incorporating some hips exercises into my yoga routine. Here are five tips for healthy hips I got from a friend, orthopedist John Corning in Chicago.

1. Stay active - even small amounts of exercise can help maintain strong muscles, slow bone loss and improve balance, keeping your hips strong and flexible. Hip flexor moves, gentle yoga and water exercises, walking and cycling all helps. Gentle yoga and water exercises supports your weight and reduces joint stress.

2. Maintain a healthy weight - For every ten pounds of extra bodyweight you carry, there's an added fifty pounds of pressure on your hips and knees.

3. Stand tall - Practicing good posture is also essential. When we stand, walk and sit in a poor posture, it puts unnecessary train and stress on the muscles supporting the hips. When standing, line your head with your shoulders and keep your shoulders directly over your hips.

4. Wear proper shoes - The shoes you wear can have a big impact. Comfortable shoes that provide the right support will improve the alignment of your joint and reduce the pressure put on them. Make sure shoes have a soft, shock-absorbing sole to reduce the impact from your feet hitting the ground.

5. Get good sleep - Using a knee pillow while sleeping each night can promote daily hip health. Without a knee pillow, the upper knee rests on the lower knee and this arrangement can

misalign the back, putting pressure on the hips and creating pain.

DEALING WITH ARTHRITIS

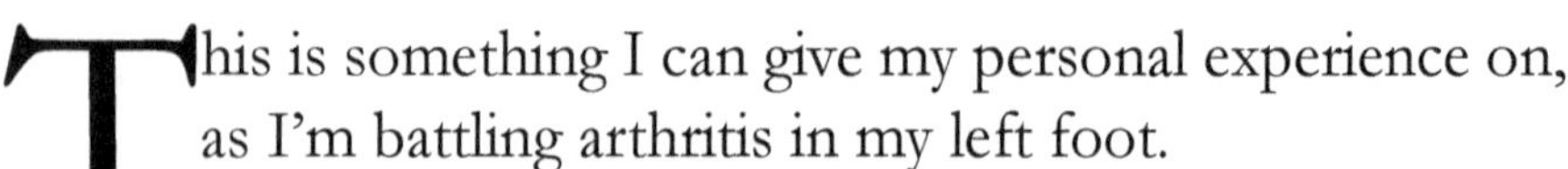

This is something I can give my personal experience on, as I'm battling arthritis in my left foot.

Osteoarthritis is one of the most common diseases among adults age 65-older, yet arthritis in general can affect those much younger and can really do a number on your feet. While we tend to associate arthritis with the knees, hips and hands, your feet and ankles actually contain about twenty-five percent of all your bones and a large number of small joints. We all know those creaky sounds that arthritic joints make. It took a visit to a conscientious podiatrist to inform me of the arthritis I had in my feet.

When you consider the daily stressful movements your feet and ankles make and the load they must routinely bear day in and day out, almost any arthritic flare-up can trigger pain and swelling. I know when I overdo it, am not getting enough rest or proper nutrition, I've more noticeably observed my arthritis symptoms once I reached my 50s. I can also tell when I've been sitting for too long.

Approximately thirty-three percent of older Americans are affected by osteoarthritis, making it the most common form of arthritis. It was believed that it was simply the result of age-related wear and tear of the joints, as well as the body failing to produce enough cartilage. Studies indicate the underlying cause is similar to that of rheumatoid arthritis, which happens when the body's immune system mistakenly attacks the cells in its joints. This leads to the release of inflammatory stuff that damages not just the cartilage, but also the bones. This disease produces a dangerous amount of inflammation that affects the rest of the body. How you manage the symptoms of arthritis over time is key to avoiding feet and overall pain and loss of mobility.

The damage from osteoarthritis in the feet can't be reversed, so the best approach is to manage it with over-the-counter medication and orthodic inserts and arch supports in the shoes. For more serious flare-ups, you may need to see your doctor for steroids or other types of injections or topical agents. If those treatments don't help and the pain becomes too severe, surgery may be required.

Exercise can help too. The pain and stiffness may improve if you get moving and stay moving. Repetitive motion is like grease for the joints and builds muscle strength. Exercise also helps reduce pain and the better you can support the joints and absorb the pressure you place on them. You just need to be careful. Lighter exercise movements like Tai Chi and yoga are other good choices, as well as aquadynamics or pool aerobics. The four components of fitness mush be attended to when dealing with arthritis - cardiovascular endurance, muscle strength, muscle endurance, flexibility training. The joints, where bones meet, and ligaments, the connective tissues which holds bones together, are affected greatly by arthritis.

This subject hits home for me as I was floored when I was told and shown the x-rays from the very patient and helpful podiatrist I had arthritis in my damaged left foot. I had a job that required lots of walking and long hours on my feet working as a quality control inspector in a health and beauty sub-contracted, manufacturing laboratory. I couldn't figure why I was in so much pain as I considered myself in pretty good shape.

There was so much swelling and pain that I had to sit from time to time during my shift. The podiatrist said all the wear and tear I've put on my feet from years of running, playing basketball, cycling, tennis and skiing/snowboarding was catching up to me.

For the first time in a long time, my mortality came into focus. The arthritis affected my circulation and caused swelling in my feet. It only came into play when I was on my feet for that long a period a time at that factory, working on those brutally hard concrete floors. It didn't help matters any I wasn't wearing the best athletic shoes for the job. My dogs were screaming for relief.

BE MINDFUL OF STIFF ANKLES

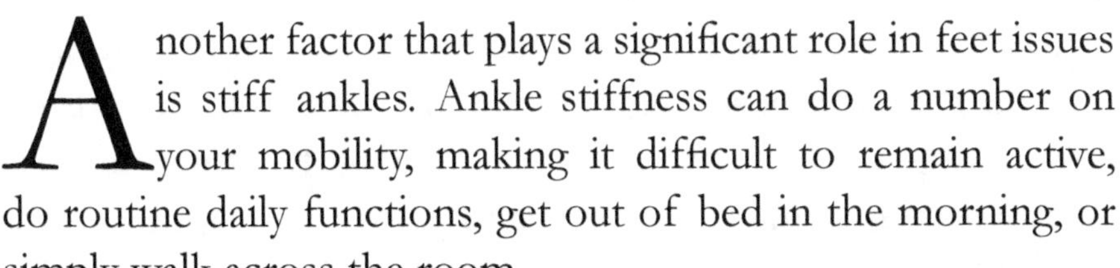

Another factor that plays a significant role in feet issues is stiff ankles. Ankle stiffness can do a number on your mobility, making it difficult to remain active, do routine daily functions, get out of bed in the morning, or simply walk across the room.

My ex-wife, who was also a personal fitness trainer, was very active and she was hampered at times having to battle her stiff ankles. I had a longtime personal training client that struggled with doing lunges and squats because of her stiff ankles. It was also tough for her to do boot camp-style exercises, especially when we were outside as running up and down hills seemed to kill her.

The ankle is a tricky joint and quite the vulnerable structure. It's made of the end of the lower leg bones (the tibia and fibula), which hold the talus bone of the foot in between them. The joint is stabilize by ligaments and powered by the muscles that work in concert in enabling ankle and feet motion and accommodating uneven surfaces when you stand or walk. If not doing well, the ankle can strain the knee, which is connected to the spine.

Ankles need flexibility. They also support and distribute your weight and that task is tougher if you are carrying extra poundage. Having your ankles supported while distributing your weight can be a tall order when you are running or jumping, which puts even more force on those joints and risks injury if it happens too much or if the foot or ankle lands the wrong way. Having strong ankles keeps you on the move for a longer period of time.

I've battled stiff ankles from around the time I started competing in baseball and basketball more seriously. It seemed like I was always spraining my ankle, most of the time the right one because as a left-handed athlete, I planted my right leg and foot as a base to generate more power and control. I was an impatient healer, often not allowing the sprain to heal before testing it again. Besides having a stress fracture I played most of my senior year of high school basketball with, I also had a nagging, high-ankle sprain that was never one hundred percent.

There are many reasons for ankle stiffness, so it's not just about age. It sucks for a lot of reasons that as we get older, but how this relates to stiff ankles - the collagen protein in our body stiffens, making soft tissues like our ligaments and tendons tighter and less resilient. That makes vulnerable joints like the ankle so much more tighter. Other conditions that can worsen age-related ankle stiffness include osteoarthritis, blood flow blockages, previous ankle injuries and persistent feet problems like flat feet or high arches that cause excessive wear on the ankles. This is why ankle mobility exercises are a must.

So what can you do for relief for stiff ankles? If it's persistently bad and doesn't seem to get better with simple exercises like ankle rolls and flexing them on a regular basis, getting massage or reflexology sessions, you might want to consider seeing a doctor to check and see if there is an inflammatory condition going on. Icing and resting your feet and ankles can help, so can physical therapy and keeping your weight under control through a healthy diet. Keeping your weight in check can help take added pressure off the ankles. Yoga, I've found, is a great antidote for stiff ankles. Often we sit too much and for too long and yoga can be like oil lubrication for suffering ankles.

One of the cooler yoga exercises I learned years ago while taking a class at Denver International Airport while I was awaiting a flight to go skiing at Aspen/Snowmass - writing the alphabet in the air with your toes while lying flat on a mat or sitting in a chair. There are a variety of chair yoga movements that are great for the feet and ankles, like just flexing your ankles up and down, to the left and to the right, as well as doing calf raises.

How you walk, sleep, run, skip, dodge is contingent on having strong ankles and this directly affects your feet too. Like I mentioned earlier, if your ankles are not functioning well that puts added stress on the knees, which are connected to the spine.

The basic foundational yoga poses, or asanas, are great for the ankles. Some of them include downward facing dog, warrior, tree and cobbler poses can do a great job of stretching and providing much needed circulation to the ankles. A great benefit of yoga is it requires proper alignment of the feet, hips and ankles to be done right. Proper hydration helps too. I've dive into more about water in another chapter, but it does have a lot to do with ankle and overall feet wellness.

✦ 46 ✦

STRETCHING

The powers of stretching overall can not be stated strongly enough. I only wish that I'd started stretching earlier in life considering how active I've been. When I talk about stretching for the feet, it really starts with stretching other parts of the body first, especially those connected to the feet.

I've mentioned how the back, shoulders, core and lower extremities all play a role in feet wellness. Not being limber and having flexibility issues can affect your posture, your overall level of comfort while bringing about pain.

Stretching your body is good for you and one of the best ways you can age gracefully and maintain being in good physical and emotional shape. However, I know many fitness-minded people who eat and exercise properly who never stretch. I didn't for years until I started having back pain and intense cramps. Stretching/flexibility is one of the main components of fitness, along with resistance and cardiovascular training and proper nutrition.

Lack of stretching can lead to low back pain, tight hamstrings, tight hip flexors and weak abdominal muscles. Consequently, not stretching those feet muscles, and there are a lot of them, can lead to sprained ankles, cramps, heel pain, strained muscles and more. Stretching can also release tension and bad energy in the body.

Just sitting and doing calf raises, circular motions with both feet, flexing your toes by swishing them in and out, can do wonders. So can taking a golf or tennis ball, putting it on the floor and rolling it all over your feet from the heels to the toes. Consider taking five minutes or so to do this when you get up in morning and when you go to bed. Of all the fitness-related things you'll probably do within the course of a day, stretching takes the less time, especially if your are focused on the feet.

You can take a few minutes to massage your feet, if you don't have an enthusiastic partner to do so. As we age, the blood flow to the feet diminishes which can make any existing feet problems worse. For example, less blood flow to a tendon in a foot could contribute to issues like tendinitis. Also, feet sensitivity declines as we age, making it more difficult for our bodies to determine how hard we're striking the ground when we walk, putting us at more risk of falls.

Stretching can help with those issues. One of the main remedies for a condition called plantar fasciitis is regular stretching of the plantar tendon in the feet. By stretching with the rolling-of-the-ball method along the tendon, you get the stimulation your foot craves while also improving mobility.

Many of my clients thought stretching was only for runners and gymnasts and I had to let them know it's something that needs to be done on a regular basis to keep muscles flexible, strong and healthy, which helps range of motion in joints and tendons. Sitting too much causes tight hamstrings and being hunched over a computer a lot can do a number on your back.

It's my opinion the areas critical for mobility are in your lower extremities - your calves, hamstrings, hip flexors and quads, as it relates to your feet. There are no quick fixes and you'll have to do this over time. It may have taken you a lifetime to get tight muscles so getting flexible won't happen overnight.

To be in top shape you need to spend equal amounts of time with flexibility, proper nutrition, cardiovascular and resistance training. Often the back pain that people get comes from tight hamstrings and hip flexor muscles, along with weak abdominal muscles. And just stretching to your maximum shouldn't be the goal here, just go for that feeling of loosening your muscles. Actually, of the four mentioned pillars of fitness, flexibility requires the least amount of time, say five to ten minutes in the morning and evening, or about 15 minutes at the end of a workout. I do yoga and stretching for approximately 20-30 minutes, five times a week, sometimes the sessions are longer on the afternoons I don't do cardiovascular work or weight training.

Don't let age be the deciding factor as to whether you stretch or not. Either you do or you don't. You can get away with not paying attention to flexibility for a while, but it will catch up with you eventually. I consistently saw this with weekend athletes who went at it hard without properly stretching and warming up before or after their chosen activity.

Flexibility can decline as we age and raise your risk of injury. We become less limber, muscles shrink and tendons also lose their water content, which makes the body stiffer.

This lack of flexibility can really make everyday movements involving the feet and lower extremities such as walking up stairs or squatting difficult. Main train spots - the hips, legs and lower back - all have an impact on the feet.

One of my favorite yoga moves is downward facing dog, which targets the back, hamstrings and calves. You are on all fours with hands should-width apart, legs hip-width apart and you are in an upside-down "V", keeping everything in alignment and pressing heels down toward the floor while keeping shoulders down and rolled back, if you need to bend knees.

I read a recent study that indicated about eighty percent of Americans suffer lower back pain at some point in their life because of tight hamstrings, tight hip flexors and weak abdominal muscles. Pilates, I've found, can help, focusing on the core to gain strength for the entire body.

GUT HEALTH AS IT RELATES TO YOUR FEET

Bloat is not just restricted to our bellies, although it often starts there. Our digestive system plays a key role in our overall health, impacting how we feel and function. Our gut acts like a second brain and that brain and our gut live together. A complex and sophisticated nervous system called the enteric nervous system, contains more than 100 million nerve cells that line our GI tract.

An unhealthy gut can cause inflammation that can cause skin problems and a failure to heal from feet problems such as Athlete's Feet and plantar fasciitis quickly. An unhealthy gut can be the cause of weight gain, which puts more pressure on your feet, back, legs and may play a role in arthritis.

Lacking those healthy microbiomes in your gut can also lead to an overactive immune system. Additionally, poor gut health can lead to poor overall circulation, especially in the feet. Certain foods cause gas, makes you feel heavy and lethargic, which can result in you looking heavier than you are. Major culprits include sugar, salt, processed foods, alcohol and smoking.

It can be prudent to aim for a plant-based diet that's low in fat. This encourages the growth of good bacteria with prebiotic and probiotic foods. Prebiotic foods include apples, asparagus, bananas, broccoli, garlic, lentils, oats, onions, honey and cabbage. Probiotic foods have gotten plenty of notoriety in recent years as it relates to overall health in general and gut health specifically. Examples include the fermented drink Kefir, kimchi, pickles, yogurt and apple cider vinegar.

When I started doing high-intensity interval training, but at the same time wasn't consuming the most effective foods beforehand, I noticed a drop in my energy and that affected my workouts. Once I educated myself and started to consume more prebiotic and probiotic foods, I noticed less bloating, better regularity and more stamina.

Other foods to help beat the bloat that should help produce healthier feet include citrus fruits (metabolism boosting), nuts and seeds (healthy fiber), watermelon (high-water fruit to flush you out) and cinnamon (for maintaining and lowering blood sugar levels).

Stress and medication can also be the cause of a poor gut. Drinking lots of water and consuming those high-water content foods will help flush your body out. Make sure you get some form of moderate exercise for at least thirty minutes each day.

Many of the problems associated with feet issues stem from bloating. Not just bloating of the feet, but also the knees, ankles, calves and legs. Many people think bloating is the result of something simple, but many body issues and often joint pain in the feet can be directly tied to bloating.

As I mentioned earlier, there are many causes such as drinking too much alcohol and other empty calorie beverages, dehydration, constipation, depression, night eating, not getting enough daily fiber, a sedentary lifestyle and consuming too much processed foods and salt are some of the factors.

These problematic issues cause inflammation, poor circulation, extra weight on the body and a slower metabolism.

Bloat can be painful and cause joint pain resulting in osteoarthritis and balance issues. An extra ten pounds of weight puts thirty to sixty more pounds of force on the knees, for example.

We need to unlock the blood vessels so they can expand, increasing blood flow and when this flow is gut off, the result can be bloating of the hands, legs and feet.

To sum it all up, the solution to any gut problem is simple. Build meals around fiber-rich foods, drink plenty of fluids and add some fermented foods to your diet. Feeding your gut well can result in losing weight, you'll have a stronger lining, you will sleep better, think more sharply, ease a troubled belly and overall just feel better.

On balance

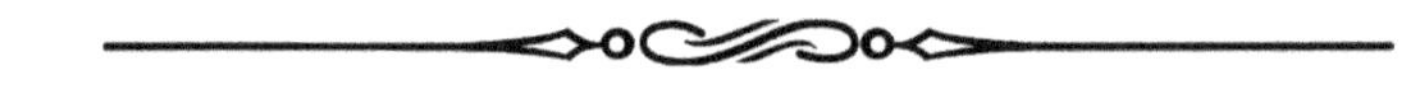

I've had a friend for years who's been very active and is youthful for her age, yet in recent years she's had balance issues.

One of the more unfortunate things that comes with aging can be balance problems. My friend confided in me it was scary for her one day when as she was putting on her bicycle shorts for a 25-mile trek, she struggled getting them on one leg at a time without shaking and wobbling trying to balance on one leg.

Professionals I've talked to about this agree that unfortunately balance declines with age and even though you can be perfectly healthy in other aspects of your life, you can still struggle with balance. Balance involves the body's ability to maintain equilibrium while standing or moving. You are coordinating your sensory system to maintain balance. You want to have static balance, being able to stand in a stationary position, and dynamic balance, being able to maintain balance during body movements.

I've dealt with this as a personal fitness trainer helping folks suffering serious consequences as a result of declining balance. Fractures, sprains and pulled muscles are just some of the unfortunate results for someone losing their overall balance.

Every year, more than one in four older Americans fall, according to the Centers for Disease Control and Prevention, with nearly three million treated annually in emergency departments for fall-related injuries. In 2022, over 30,000 folks aged 65-older died as a result of falls. One in four seniors have a serious fall resulting in an emergency room visit. According to the American Association for Retired People, by 2030 59,000 seniors will have died as the result of a fall. Hearing loss, social isolation and loneliness are major contributors to balance struggles.

Falls due to balance are more common in the elderly and can lead to fractures, especially hip fractures. Woman with osteoporosis for example, may never be the same again after a fall related to balance.

People of any age can have balance-related issues, which can be caused by health conditions, medications or problems in the inner ear or the brain. Symptoms of balance disorders can include dizziness or vertigo, lightheadedness, blurred vision or disorientation.

So how do you deal with balance concerns? Aerobic workouts, strength training, stretching and specific exercises aimed at improving balance are all good. One of my favorite things to do for balance is yoga and one of my favorite poses is called tree pose, where you stand alternately on one leg with the other one bent with your foot resting on your shin, calf or inner thigh of the standing leg, with your hands resting at your heat in a prayer position or held above your head like you are a football official signaling a touchdown.

Balance as it relates to feet can involve many issues such as poor posture, back pain, weakened muscles and feet problems such as corns, bunions, heel pain and poor circulation. Getting too much salt, or not enough water can also be contributing factors related to your feet that can affect your balance.

Stretching, having a good diet as being overweight and putting too much pressure on your feet can affect balance too, and strengthening your feet through yoga and resistance training can greatly help you deal with balance issues related to your feet. The same goes for wearing supportive and the right kind of shoes.

People need to understand there is a relationship between balance and strength, another reason to incorporate some exercises into your day. These exercises don't have to take up a lot of your time either. The following are some good and easy ones I recommend.

1. Toe tap - Standing with one hand on a wall for stability, keep both legs straight, lift one leg and stretch it in front of you until its at forty-five degrees from your body, toes pointed, then touch toes to the ground, hold a moment, then do again.

2. Bodyweight squats - from different angles.

3. Tree pose - In this yoga posture raise on leg and place foot on inside of other leg, either on ankle, calf, skin or inner thigh, place hands in a prayer position near your heart or arms raised above your head and hold for a few seconds before repeating with other leg.

4. Sitting in a chair - flexing your toes up and down, your ankles up and down and from side to side and just curling your toes and squeezing and releasing them.

5. Simply marching in walking in place.

6. Do standing calf stretches.

7. Bridges.

8. Hip flexor stretch.

9. Standing side leg lifts.

10. Standing on one leg at a time for about thirty seconds each.

There are thirty-three bones in the feet and its scary how poor balance can lead to many feet issues. We need core stability, strong legs, back, ankles and feet. As we age, the disks in our back shorten and there is more curvature in the spine. We need to sit less, do more flexibility training like yoga and general stretching, core and resistance training, have your vision and hearing checked regularly, wear the right shoes and focus hard on lubricating those feet and ankles. These are great preventative measures to take to maintain good balance as we age.

Pay attention when walking down the street and notice how some people seem to move about out of balance. It's more prevalent than you think. Maintaining balance as you age is serious stuff. The business of balance needs to be approached like a job. There are over two hundred connective tissue disorders that in some way affect balance. We need more balance work than we think - like working on hips and posture, freeing blockage from the connective tissue network.

We are hunched over computers, cell phones and have rounded backs. Balance, core and stability training are main components of my fitness world. I remember how eye-opening it was for me when I first started doing yoga and was in lying relaxation pose on a yoga mat and noticed the difference in balance between the left side of my body and the right. I had no idea I had been working with such an imbalance.

A WORD ABOUT SALT

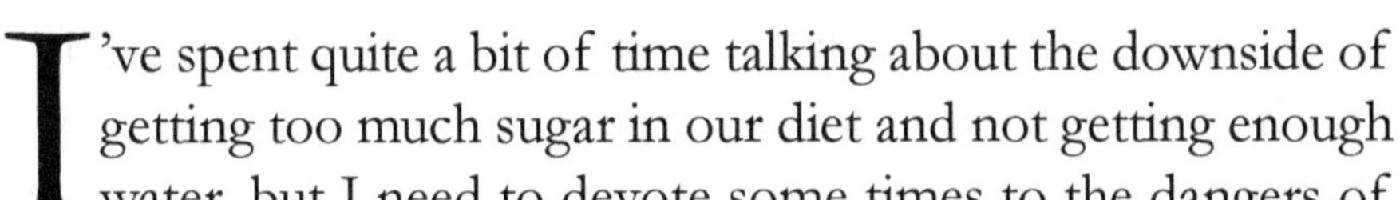

I've spent quite a bit of time talking about the downside of getting too much sugar in our diet and not getting enough water, but I need to devote some times to the dangers of getting too much sodium.

The average person in this country gets way too much salt. The amount we should get should be roughly be the equivalent of one teaspoon daily. There is so much salt hidden in foods and ninety percent of us gets an abundance. The excess sodium in the body leads to puffiness and bloating.

Salt is in abundance in restaurant foods - a reason why more cravings equal more profits and that extra salt can encourage us to drink more, a big things coveted by restaurant owners. Little did I know all the times I was eating at places like Applebee's and TGI Fridays that I was getting many days worth of sodium in my delicious meals.

Surprisingly, breakfast foods, baked goods like breads and even vegetable juices carry more sodium than you realize. Even so-called healthy foods like boneless chicken breasts can be plumped up with a salt and water solution to make them more visually appealing at the grocery store. And just think of all the salt that goes into your marinades.

Salt can dry out your skin and again too much of it can make you look and feel dehydrated and contribute to high blood pressure. Our feet are susceptible to dry skin anyway, so having too much sodium in our diets can make dry skin issues with our feet even worse.

Besides taking it easy with salt and staying away from processed foods, which are loaded with sodium, here are some other ways to eliminate salt from your diet.

1. Eat foods rich in potassium. Not only does bananas, avocados and spinach help with cramps and sore muscles, they also help break down the sodium intake in our bodies.

2. Try low sodium salt.

3. Add some smoke flavoring to food instead, like paprika.

4. Try spicy flavors like cayenne pepper.

5. Add an acid to your food, like lemon, apple cider vinegar or white wine vinegar. I love a mixture of lemon zest, parsley and garlic instead of salt on many of the foods I eat.

6. Drink lots of water - about half your weight in ounces of water daily.

It's hard because salt is everywhere. Trying to live a life of wellness should include some mindfulness effort paid to keeping our overall sodium numbers in check. Most of us eat more than 3,500 milligrams of salt daily. The American Heart Association says we should only have around 2,300 milligrams daily if we are healthy and only 1,500 milligrams a day for older adults, people of color and those having high blood pressure, diabetes or kidney issues.

The salt we consume is sodium chloride and it's made up of forty percent sodium and sixty percent chloride. We actually do need salt in our bodies to survive, but when we get too much of it, our bodies hold extra water to flush the salt away, which raises blood volume, can lead to high blood pressure and kidney and heart disease because the kidneys and the heart have to work harder. Having too much salt in you can negatively affect your workout if you are not properly hydrated. I've seen people who eat a lot of processed and fast food that had consistent swelling in their feet, making walking and exercising uncomfortable.

Here are some other sodium-reducing tips to consider:

1. Read food labels and cut down on your consumption of take out and fast food.

2. Choose frozen over canned vegetables, which can contain a lot of sodium.

3. Leave all those salty potato and snack chips alone.

4.Watch out for spice blends, which can have hidden salt.

5.Remember that low fat doesn't mean low salt. Salt is sometimes added for flavor.

6. Get rid of the salt shaker so you won't be tempted.

7. Look for low sodium choices in food and drinks.

Watching your sodium intake is one of easier things you can do to help your feet look and feel healthy.

DEALING WITH FLAT FEET

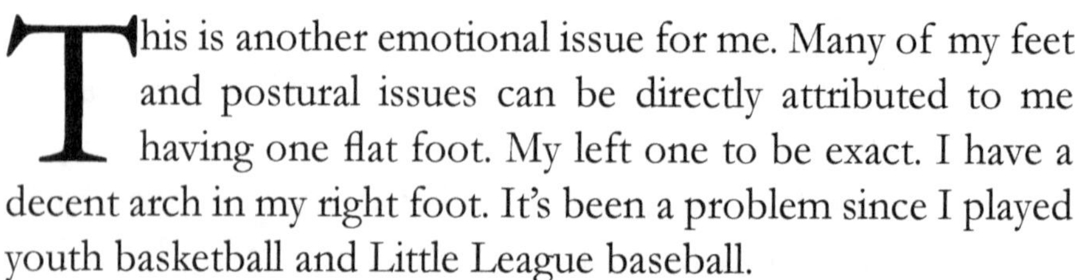

This is another emotional issue for me. Many of my feet and postural issues can be directly attributed to me having one flat foot. My left one to be exact. I have a decent arch in my right foot. It's been a problem since I played youth basketball and Little League baseball.

It was confusing to me that my back bothered me all of the time and I found out in later years that one leg was a few centimeters shorter than the other. I still to this day walk with the slightest of limbs, particularly when I'm tired.

Flat feet occur over time because of fatigue in the supporting tendons, ligaments and soft tissues of the feet. This causes the arch to collapse, so the sole of the feet comes in contact with the ground, or close to it. While this often is the result of many years of wear and tear on the feet, in my case it was genetic. Both my mom and grandmother had flat feet.

Having flat feet is a tough problem to tackle for a typical person, let alone an active one like myself. Your arches can become painful and your feet can tire easily. I somewhat built up a tolerance for the pain I had in my one flat foot from a life span full of sports and fitness activities, but it slowly got worse as I aged. Like me, your gait or stance may change, you may experience leg and/or back pain as your body tries to compensate for the imbalance caused by one or two flat feet.

You can have balance issues - mine came when I started running long distances. Flat feet can cause havoc for some in job settings, for those on their feet all day like coaches or someone in the hospitality industry.

You can do a simple check to see if you have flat feet. Wet your feet then stand on a flat surface that will show your footprint. Flat feet typically reveal an outline of the entire bottom of the foot as opposed to just part of the front and back.

Unfortunately when it comes to family history, flat feet are not preventable. If the condition is caused by aging, there are ways to strengthen and support your arches and slow down the progression of the arch collapse. Something to keep in mind, our feet flatten out as we age and it is not uncommon even for those without flat feet becoming a shoe size larger than they were years ago.

I have a friend who insisted on forcing her aging and flattening feet into the same size nine shoes even though she admitted her shoes felt a bit uncomfortable. Over time she damaged her big toenails to the point they had to be removed. There had been too much pressure on them for too long a time. She said her doctor initially noticed some discoloration in her nails.

Some tips for dealing with flat feet:

1. Use over-the-counter or custom orthodics.

2. Wear supportive shoes.

3. Engage in exercises for the calves, feet, ankles and hamstrings.

4.Limit high-impact or repetitive activities and switch to low impact ones, like going from running to walking or cycling instead of hiking when you experience feet pain.

5. Invest in a pair of compression socks.

6.Consider getting massage, reflexology or acupressure sessions.

7. Soak feet in warm, swirling water, which can help with pain and circulation.

8. Consider getting a treadmill instead of walking outside as the treadmill has more give to it.

9. Get a tennis or golf ball and roll it over your flat feet, heels and balls of your feet as this can help with overall circulation.

10. Apply ice packs and elevate feet to ease swelling and discomfort.

11. Try walking around barefoot - this can strengthen feet and help them naturally realign.

12. Do exercises such as squats, lunges, calf raises and certain yoga poses that target the lower body like tree and warrior pose.

13. Avoid wearing pointed or high heels if you are standing for long periods. These are killers for flat feet.

14, Choose shoes with good arch support.

15. Avoid wearing thick, stiff shoes as they affect flexibility.

16. Make sure your shoes fit well, leaving enough room in the toe box, at least one-half an inch.

17. Maintain toenail health - this could help reduce trauma and create extra room in shoes. You'll also reduce the risk of nail breakage, which can provide a port of entry for fungus.

18. Keep feet cool and dry.

19. Take a short walk break at work to stretch those muscles.

20. Standup and stretch, or walk in place at your work station.

TRY REFLEXOLOGY AND AROMATHERAPY FOR FEET PAIN

Back in ancient times, shoes were unknown properties and people walked around barefoot over all types of terrain with the reflex zones of the feet (areas that reflect images of places in the body) getting stimulated on a regular basis, so there was no need for reflexology. Feet issues are so severe today, as we cram our feet into fashionable, toe-crunching athletic and high-heeled shoes leading to arthritis, corns, hammer toes, bunions and an assortment of other problems.

Some women's shoe styles often don't allow enough room for the feet to expand (as the result of being involved in endurance sports, having their period or simply getting too much salt). I worked at a specialty athletic shoe store once and remember getting into battles with customers when I suggested they considered purchasing larger shoe sizes to help protect their feet. Most of these conversations were with women. And it's not just with active people, folks in all walks of life are subjected to feet injuries and having a vast array of solutions is a prudent thing.

This is where reflexology comes in and giving a session a try might help. I admit I was skeptical when it was suggested to me after running a 10-kilometer race once and I had intense pain afterwards. Reflexology has some of the same benefits as massage in that it induces stress and provides a deep relaxation and also can help alleviate pain.

So how does it work? Well, it promises to relieve feet tension and clear blockages by stimulating sensory receptors in the nerve fibers of the feet, producing energy that branches to the spinal cord where its dispersed throughout the entire nervous system. It also helps with circulation. Opinions vary, but the six or seven times I've had a reflexology session it worked wonders on my tired and aging feet and I asked other clients who tried it as well and they said they got relief.

I try to simply break it down and tell people reflexology is simply the application of applying appropriate pressure to specific points and areas of the feet. For example, reflexology holds a belief that a specific spot in the arch of the foot corresponds to the bladder. When a reflexologist uses thumbs or fingers to manipulate this area, it can affect bladder functioning. In a way, its similar to acupuncture and acupressure in that it works with the body's vital energy.

I first got introduced to reflexology and aromatherapy several years ago stopping by booths at health and fitness expositions in Chicago. I initially thought both modalities were bogus.

Months later, working on a story for *American Fitness* magazine on alternative healing therapies, my research led me to trying both reflexology and aromatherapy. The experiences, along with getting to know several practitioners, completely changed my perspective.

Reflexology is basically the application of applying appropriate pressure to specific points and areas of the feet, hands or ears. Practitioners believe these areas and reflex points correspond to different organs and systems and that manipulating them has a beneficial effect on the organs and the person's overall health.

For example, reflexology holds that a specific spot in the arch of the foot corresponds to the bladder. When a reflexologist uses thumbs or fingers to apply appropriate pressure to this area, it affects bladder functioning. This is similar to acupuncture and acupressure in that it works with the body's vital energy through stimulation of points in the body. Sometimes people confuse it with massage, which works from the outside in, as opposed to reflexology working from the inside out.

Aromatherapy is the art of blending essential oils extracts distilled from aromatic flavors, plants, herbs or fruits for the purposes of restoring balance to the mind, body and spirit. For example, putting lavender oil on the temples is said to help ease headaches. Basil oil is said to stimulate the brain and rosemary oil is said to be a great memory drug, with sage being a tonic for mental fatigue. The smells supposedly connects with sensors in our brain. Some of the other more popular essential oils include citrus oils, almond oil, tea tree and peach-kernel oil.

Worst case, both treatments are relaxing and many people I've interviewed have found both modalities helpful. Both have also been used to compliment other treatments for anxiety, asthma, diabetes, PMS and kidney function.

For those who can't afford professional treatments, practitioners have provided me all the information to do self treatments at home. I would say leave the aromatherapy treatments to the experts who know firsthand how to deal with essential oils.

An aromatherapy session will include a practitioner dabbing a cotton ball with an essential oils such as peppermint and requesting that the patient inhale like he or she was smelling a flower, then exhale like they were blowing out a candle.

Essential oils have become a big deal in today's holistic healing world, being promoted as a natural way to improve mood, ward off sickness and treat ailments such as dry skin, arthritis and allergies, although research on the benefits is not conclusive.

The essential oil are now more mainstream and can be found in grocery stores, as well as online.

I equate aromatherapy similar to that feeling you get when you smell a peeled orange or sniff real vanilla. It promotes a positive feeling. I can see how it could provide quick relief from depression and anxiety. Again, I personally find that both treatments work.

Sometimes aromatherapy and reflexology sessions are combined. The smells can put you in the right mental space for a reflexology session, which again really does differ from traditional massage. There are so many pressure points in the feet and all that poking, toe twisting, ankle flexing and heel work that goes into a reflexology session does provide relief.

FROM A REFLEXOLOGISTS' POINT OF VIEW

One of the big things that comes from having a reflexologist as a personal training client is the knowledge they can provide. My client Krista use to always preach to me how your health was truly connected to your joints, hands and feet. She spent a lot of time in hand and feet study and analysis and said your palms can reveal how you are feeling, your general state of health and even if you are pre-disposed to a particular condition. I remember seeing women who specialized in Chinese medicine telling me the same things years earlier and how at the time I thought that was garbage.

For example, Krista said discoloration in nails often is often a sign of nutritional deficiency, how rough hands can be a sign of dehydration and soft hands a sign of an active metabolism. She said healthy looking nails and good nail growth are signs you're getting enough nutrition, hydration and physical stimulation.

"Poor diet, inactivity and inflammation are easy to see, you can tell the age, health and a lot about a person by looking at their hands and feet," she said.

Other reflexology wisdom, according to Krista Cunningham:

1. The brain and sinus are connected to the big toes.

2. The neck, eyes and ears are connected to the areas just under the toes.

3. The thyroid, lungs and heart are connected to the balls of your feet.

4. The spine, lumbar and bladder are connected to the edge of your feet under the big toes.

5. The stomach and pancreas are connected to the middle foot.

6. The small intestine and sciatic nerves and pelvic are connected to the middle foot and heels.

7. The knee and hips are connected to the edge of the foot.

HOW POOR POSTURE CAN AFFECT YOUR FEET

Because of my alignment and foot issues, I had poor posture long before I ever knew what poor posture was. Many people I've noticed in various walks of life struggle with poor posture for a variety of reasons. Sometimes it's a hereditary thing, more often their poor posture is the result of a variety of factors such as a weak back, weak core muscles or other feet concerns.

Maintaining good posture and alignment is one of my passions since it has been a struggle to maintain for most of my life. My one leg is only centimeters shorter than the other, but combining that factor with a flat and poorly-healed injured left foot, resulted in my body trying to compensate and one negative ending result was poor posture.

So what is good posture and what does that have to do with feet? Posture is the position in which you hold your body upright against gravity while standing, sitting or lying down. Good posture involves training your body to stand, walk, sit and lie in positions where the least strain is placed on supporting muscles and ligaments during movement or weight-bearing activities. Proper posture keeps bones and joints in correct alignment so the muscles are used properly, preventing backache and muscle pain, helping decrease the changes of arthritis and contributing to a good overall appearance.

If your feet are hurting, you wear shoes with poor support, wear high heels often, do a lot of running and walking, these tings can affect the way you stand. Sometimes, our posture is compromised as we compensate for feet pain while we walk or sit. Shoes wear out. Age, a poor diet and lifestyle can also contribute to poor posture. Issues with posture definitely can affect your feet.

Luckily, even if you have the worst posture in the world there are things that you can do to help take some of the pressure off your back and consequently your feet.

1. Stand and sit with your back straight and shoulders back and avoid sitting or standing in the same position for more than thirty minutes at a time.

2. Engage in resistance training, paying attention to working your shoulders, back, core and legs. Poor posture is often the result of de-conditioned muscles. Particular exercises like squats, calf raises and lunges are good for the strength and circulation of the feet, as well as many yoga poses like downward dog and the one-legged tree pose.

3. Stretch - From your feet up to your back. Stiff and tight muscles can be a major contributor to posture problems. Make a concentrated effort to try and relax those muscles that have been in a locked position.

4.Stay hydrated - A lack of water can contribute to among other things, stiff muscles and a lack of energy that could result in you not placing your body in the proper alignment zone.

5. Try alternative therapies - Like yoga, reflexology and different types of massage. The low back pain leading to feet pain can be dealt with through a wide variety of modalities.

6. Invest in an exercise ball - It's a great piece of equipment that if used right can provide some exercises to help deal with posture-related pain. Spine extensions. Pelvic tilts, bridges and lumbar extensions are a few exercises that can be executed using a ball.

7.Walk - Perhaps the easiest and cheapest way to deal with posture issues is to walk mindfully with shoulders back, the back straight and your head in a neutral position. Walking helped me with my posture and feet issues - my feet got stronger.

8. Keeping a healthy weight - Feet, back and other bodyparts are affected by carrying around extra weight, which puts added strain on muscles. Our feet take enough pounding as it is without adding extra pounds to our frame.

9. Invest in the right shoes - They should have good support, be checked regularly for uneven wear. Avoid being in high heels for long periods of time.

10. Maintain good feet health - Corns, bunions, plantar fasciitis and other issues can make you compromise the way you walk, resulting in poor posture. See a podiatrist once in a while.

11. Get creative - I enlisted the help of several postural therapists that provided me some exercises. Sit and stand ten times with a chair behind you. Do ankle rolls, lie on your back with one leg straight and make twenty ankle circles in each direction, then point and flex the toes twenty times before

repeating with the other ankle. Then try static back, when you lie on your back with hips and knees bent at ninety degrees with your lower legs resting on the seat of the chair. Extend your arms out to the side with palms up. Hold this for five minutes.

I'm quite passionate about posture work and the role it plays in feet health. Because of my issues, like I said I've struggled with maintaining proper posture. It took a combination of core work, stronger back and shoulder muscles, yoga and stretching to get me right and any problems with the feet puts proper posture in limbo.

Just because we are aging doesn't mean we have to have posture issues. The biggest things is making sure we don't lose muscle strength. It was so exciting to me seeing so many women at my grandmother's assistant living facility sign up for the strength training for seniors class I taught there, at the urging of my nanny. I saw so many people either sitting all the time at a computer, sitting watching television, barely moving at all. Muscles atrophy sits in with all that inactivity.

I also want to re-emphasize how important simple, regular yoga asandas (poses) can help with offering stability and aid in correcting posture. Yoga doesn't have to be taxing or difficult. I can think back to having horrible posture in high school and that putting such a strain on my back and I had no clue as to why I had so much pain. Bad posture can affect your mood too.

This was also a tough pill for me to swallow because younger people are suppose to be steadier on their feet and have strong upper bodies, particularly if you are an athlete. There is something called embodies cognition, where the brain and body live in the state you move or hold yourself in. This has an impact on your emotions and mental state.

Another posture-related dilemma - many of us sit in chairs that are either too soft or too deep and that can lead to pain and bad posture.

I look at posture as among other things the business of balance. It's hard to be productive long-term in the hospitality industry, where I worked for years, when your posture is out of whack with poor body balance. There are more than two hundred connective tissue disorders and spa workers are typically hunched over computers or phones, bent over in chairs or contorting their bodies from side to side. Poor posture can be so uncomfortable, but can be improved over time with mindfulness and a few other remedies like walking barefoot, which can reduce inflammation and pain in the knees and lower back. Other common postural problems include a sway back, a hollow back, a flat pelvis, slumping posture, military posture, rounded shoulders and forward heels.

Having knee problems can affect your posture too as knee pain can decide how you walk - even more of a reason to watch your weight, stay flexible and work on building muscle in your body.

Yoga got me consistent with back stretching, chair as well as floor work. It's amazing when you start paying attention to your body you'll notice the imbalance from one side to the other. It took me about six months of consistent yoga to get my body in harmony, which in the end affected my posture. Again, posture can be approved by using a stability and/or exercise ball. A stability ball is designed to bring movement to the spine in a controlled manner. Exercises like simple bridges or hyper-extensions on the stability ball can do wonders.

Chances are the longer you ignore posture issues the worst they will get over time.

A list of posture-related exercises:

1. Squats
2. Lunges
3.Calf raises
4. Standing stability ball twists
5. Lat pulldowns
6. One-arm rows
7. Yoga bridges
8. Bridges
9. Planks
10. Hip thrusts
11. Pelvic tilts
12. Push-ups
13. Shoulder presses
14. Upright rows

The key is to incorporate exercises that work the whole body as being in total harmony is a key to good posture.

WHAT YOUR CORE HAS TO DO WITH AGING FEET

I've had so many people ask me what does core maintenance have to do with the feet, as the two seemed completely unrelated.

I tell them so much of the power of your body comes from your core. A weak core can affect your back, shoulders, arms, legs and yes, your feet. Even if you have good overall cardiovascular and resistance training strength, it can help your feet in the long run to have a strong core.

Having a strong core helps cut your chances of injury. On the other hand, having a weak core can affect balance, posture, movement and overall strength, which can affect the way you walk, which can cause problems in your feet from corns, calluses and heel issues. Having a strong core can also help prevent everyday injuries that can happen from falls or simply bending over. Simply put, your core is at the center of everything.

Even doing something seemingly benign like bending over to tie your shoes engages your core muscles. As we age, we tend to have a decline in muscle strength and bone mass. Besides helping with our balance, having a solid core helps with basic spine movement.

During my many years as a personal trainer I've seen people with poor posture have feet problems. It's as if their whole body was out of alignment and since the feet take the brunt of the pressure, they suffer the most from the imbalance.

So what is your core? It's a set of muscles that mainly serves to stabilize and transfer forces between the upper and lower extremities. The twenty-nine pair of muscles of the back, stomach and hips can help you stand up straight, transfer energy and distribute your weight. All this affects your feet when walking or standing. If everything else is not in harmony, your feet get uneven pressure and wear. Think of how a car's tires suffer from the vehicle not being in proper alignment.

Working on core strength involves core work that helps you maintain a neutral spine. There are three natural curves in a healthy spine and the neutral alignment of these curves helps to protect it from overdo stress or strain. Core work involves more than just doing crunches. You need to work the deeper muscles in the inner core including the pelvic floor and transverse abdominal muscles. There are a variety of exercises to choose from and there are classes like Pilates, yoga and Crossfit that are great places to learn and start getting use to incorporating core work into your fitness routine. Pilates aids in core strength, stability, control and endurance. Different yoga modalities can help elongate core muscles, making them more flexible. There are a lot of core exercises that can be executed using a medicine ball and stability ball from sit-ups to crunches.

DEALING WITH TOENAIL FUNGUS

It's unsightly and seemingly never goes away and is a very important potential problem that can affect the appearance of your feet - unsightly toenail fungus.

Dealing with the external trauma of feet issues is just as important as dealing with the internal stuff and toenail fungus is not only unsightly, but it can be caused by a variety of reasons. Some professionals would lead you to believe the only way to get rid of toenail fungus would be through professional laser treatments, which can be expensive.

I've struggled with this and after educating myself I've experimented with some treatments I've perfected in my kitchen laboratory that I've found to be successful in getting rid of toenail fungus. I've also had family and friends try some of these treatments too and they've had varying degrees of success.

1. Try using a 50/-50 split of mouthwash and vinegar and applying with a cotton ball on the affected area around the toes two to three times a day for about a week.

2. Put Vicks Vapor Rub on the area daily. It's inexpensive and contains powerful antifungal stuff like menthol.

3. Put A&D ointment on the affected area daily. This is also good for cracked skin around and between the toes.

4. I picked this one up watching a television show - soak your feet in vinegar and hydrogen peroxide and add a couple of dental cleaner tablets too. This solution will not only get rid of the fungus but also provide a brightness to your toenails.

5. Use a combination of vitamin E and tea tree oil to the affected nails each morning. Both are antiviral and antibacterial.

These treatments need to be done on a consistent basis to be effective. Also, make sure to keep your feet moisturized and consider taking the supplements zinc, biotin (B-6), collagen and vitamin D-3. They can help treat the fungus, help darker nails get whiter, help grow them out, moisturize them while giving them strength.

If you want to take your toenail fungus treatment into the spa arena, here are three things to try.

Make a simple scrub by combining a little olive oil, salt, lemon juice and scrub on nails to treat fungus and help them look more healthy. Finish with a moisturizer.

Or a cleanser/exfoliation scrub of one tablespoon of baking soda, one-half a teaspoon of honey, one-fourth cup of reduced fat milk, one cup of salt and two tablespoons of olive oil. Mix and scrub all over affected nails and do this treatment at least two times a week until condition improves.

My friend Krista loves this simple scrub and said it worked - combining two tablespoons of honey, four tablespoons of sugar and one tablespoon of lemon juice and scrub the affected toenails. You can do this treatment several times a week.

✦ 83 ✦

DON'T NEGLECT TAKING CARE OF YOUR TOENAILS

Not taking care of your toenails can cause all sorts of feet-related issues including pain. Additionally, taking care of your feet to keep you functioning well is one thing, but many would agree they also want them to look good.

There are a myriad of reasons why someone would have dry, yellow, brittle, dark or generally unhealthy looking nails.

Poor diet is one reason, not getting enough water, not eating power foods or those foods that promote healthy circulation and not getting enough fiber and protein are other factors. Then there is consuming too much salt, sugar and fat which causes inflammation in the body and that can affect your nails. They also can raise your cholesterol numbers, which in terms affect blood flow.

Solutions? Be active as inactivity slows circulation and body metabolism in the body, more specifically in this case your feet and nails. Improve your diet, as inactivity combined with inflammation while consuming foods lacking in nutrition are other factors in bad nail health. Walking, any cardiovascular exercise, yoga, reflexology and massage are all good in bringing good blood flow to the feet and toenails.

Soak your feet and nails regularly. Use a foot basin or take a bath loaded with Epsom salt, powdered milk and oatmeal for example. All are loaded with good stuff for the skin and nails. Feet and toenails can get bacteria easily.

Or you can try a favorite feet soak of mine where you put green tea, olive oil, lemon slices and apple cider vinegar in a feet basin or whirlpool foot bath. Both of these can get rid of external issues like dry skin and fungus while also making your feet and nails look more healthy.

Older people tend to have more problems with their nails and sometimes they don't have the flexibility or dexterity to bend down or tend to them as much.

Cracked, brittle toenails may come from fungus infection, or you've cut them wrong, banged the toe or toes on something hard and damaged them. People with less circulation also tend to have more problems with their toenails.

I'm a big fan of supplements. Biotin and most of the B vitamins help with hair, skin and nails, the same goes with collagen. The supplement zinc helps with overall body metabolism. Calcium and vitamin D-3 helps with nail health. Omega-3 fatty acids aid in circulation, the same with vitamin E. At a minimum, take a daily multi-vitamin.

I came across something that among other things helped in aiding the repair I had from a damaged toenail - toega. It's a real thing, basically it's yoga for your toes that helps with flexibility and blood flow and good blood flow is like medicine for a damaged toenail.

THE POWER OF TREATMENTS FOR YOUR FEET

With my old age and experience, I've found myself to be a big fan of treatments. Many of the places here I either experienced treatments or got the inspiration to try new ones came from several vacation-based spas I've visited during my travels over the years.

Some of them:

The Spa at the Four Seasons Hotel in Toronto

The Spa at Copper Mountain Resort in Colorado

Spa NaLai at the Park Hyatt Hotel in New York City

The Salamander Resort and Spa in Middleburg, Virginia

Mohawk Mountain House in New Paltz, New York

Naly Kinetic Spa at Turtle Bay Resort in Hawaii

The Spa at Canyon Ranch Resort in Arizona

Alana's Day Spa in Chicago

Space Time Tanks in Chicago

I've picked the minds of many salon owners, workers, nail technicians, aestheticians, reflexologists and other body care providers who've been extremely helpful in supplying meaningful intelligence. I was also fortunate enough to have family member and a personal training client working in the industry who was somewhat of an expert in all natural treatments for the body.

The interest in treatments was also sparked from an assignment given to me by a health and fitness magazine I did freelance writing for. They wanted me a write a piece on ways spa/health care and hospitality workers could extend the life of their careers by taking care of their feet from the physical and cosmetic benefits. It was from all the research and interviews I did for this story running in *DaySpa Magazine* that I learned of many of the powers of non-medical treatments and combing this with my own personal experience I figured out the importance of taking care of your feet from a professional perspective. The completed story made me hungry for more information.

I have to admit I was hooked after getting my first pedicure that included a citrus-based, exfoliation scrub.

The cool thing is you don't have to go to a high-end, expensive spa to experience the benefits of a good treatment and you can save money by using ingredients at home. Natural stuff like lemons, berries, sugar and oils work great.

I was due to start a new job when COVID-19 hit, so starting the new job got delayed which gave me the time to create and experiment in my kitchen remedies for my stress-related eczema. I was so tired dealing with the painful, dry, cracked and red skin on my face and feet.

The following are some very simple home face treatments that also can be used on the feet.

These treatments will have to stay on you for 15-20 minutes for them to work. I was inspired by a face and hands treatment I got while at Whistler and Blackcomb Resort in British Columbia, Canada while there for a ski excursion. Just like with most all natural treatments, using fruits provides vitamins antioxidants, salt and sugar serves as exfoliate, honey works as an anti-bacterial/anti-inflammatory, with eggs and yogurt helping to brighten and tighten the skin. Oils provide the moisture.

Some of my male friends have given me a hard time for being into facials, but I tell them I do what I can to slow down the aging process. The following are some of the facial treatments I initially tried with success and then tried them on my feet because the eczema on my feet was typically worse than on my face and I wanted to try something different from what I typically used.

Blueberry - smash one cup of blueberries and mix with one-half cup of olive oil and two egg whites.

Sweet potato - put one baked sweet potato, two tablespoons of lemon juice and one egg in a food processor or blender.

Grapefruit - scoop out segments of one pink grapefruit, one cup of spinach, one-half cup of chia seeds and one tablespoon of lime. Blend together.

Coconut - mix one-half a cup of coconut oil, two tablespoons each of lemon juice and green tea with one tablespoon of honey and blend.

Most people are surprised to know that many of the facial treatments people use help provide hydration and nutrients to the feet as well.

There are so many medical and physical issues affecting your feet including sprains, arthritis, fungi, infections, warts, flat feet, bunions, corns, calluses, blisters, plantar fasciitis, eczema and varicose veins. Many of them will require professional help, however there are quite a bit of natural and immediate things you can do to treat certain irritations and pains. I got tired of products in stores and even prescription items that didn't cure my Athlete's Feet or eczema. I've tried the most expensive lotions and creams before I got exposed to do-it-yourself scrub treatments using all natural ingredients.

You need salt and sugar to exfoliate, a moisturizer of some kind like tea tree oil or olive oil and an antibacterial/antiviral like honey, citrus or berries. The following is five of some of my favorite general scrub treatments specifically designed to treating feet issues. Let mixture sit on feet for a few minutes before exfoliating.

Coconut/mango - mix one-half cup of coconut sugar and mango, one-third a cup of grapeseed oil and scrub on feet before washing off.

Honey/lemon - use one-fourth a cup of honey, half a cup of sugar, baking soda and lemon juice and scrub well, especially between the toes.

Aloe vera - mix one cup of salt, one-fourth a cup of olive oil, lemon juice and aloe vera gel.

Green tea - make one cup of green tea, drink half of it, mix the other half with one cup of Epsom salt, one-forth cup of almond oil and one-fourth a cup of lemon juice.

Epsom salt - use one cup of Epsom salt, one half a cup of sugar, one fourth a cup of olive oil and lemon juice.

Here are five more specific treatments for your feet.

Make bath fizzes for tired feet and to help with dry skin by combining one cup of baking soda, one-half a cup of Epsom salt, one-half a cup of regular salt, one-half a cup of lemon juice, one-half a cup of olive oil and one-fourth a cup of vanilla extract, mix together and pack down individually into ice cube trays and let sit for about 24 hours, then plop several of them into the tub for a healing bath that's sure to energize your feet.

Make a citrus scrub to wear down those calluses on your feet by taking one smashed orange, one cup of salt and one-half a cup of olive oil and scrub on the affected area.

Give those sore and unsightly cuticles a break by soaking them in foot basin of several cups of apple cider vinegar, two eggs and a cup of pineapple juice. The acid will help soften the cuticles.

You can give your dull and damaged toenails a bit of a facelift by combing one cup of green tea, one egg white, one cup of milk and one-half a cup of olive oil, mix solution and take a cotton ball and spread over your toenails, let sit for about 15-20 minutes before washing off.

Create a feet and nail exfoliation with one cup of smashed pineapple, one cup of salt, half a cup of olive oil and aloe vera gel and seriously scrub feet and toenails.

HOW TO DO AN EASY AT-HOME PEDICURE

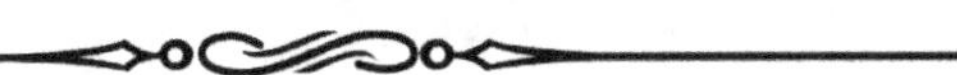

What would writing a book about taking care of your feet be without at least giving a little nod to how simple it is to give yourself a pedicure, You can eat right, keep your weight in check, exercise and see professionals when needed, but at the end of the day you do want good looking feet and toes. I was fortunate enough to have a personal training client who worked as a nail technician who owned her own salon in Chicago who provided me this easy to follow tutorial for giving yourself a basic pedicure.

1.Soak feet in water for at least twenty minutes and then wash them well. For yellow nails, drop a few denture-cleaning tablets in the water before soaking, or even apple cider vinegar.

2. Dry your feet well and use a nail file to correct any imperfections in the nails.

3. Massage them with a gritty exfoliation scrub.

4. Apply a base coat followed by two layers of polish.

5. Let pedicure rest for at least thirty minutes.

6. Use a good quality moisturizer once nails dry.

Beware of aging feet as well as hands. Although hands show aging more than any other bodypart and the feet often age the less than say the hands or face, they still age. Feet are subject to agents that dry them out like water, ultra violet rays and extreme temperatures. As we age the skin on our feet dries out and the toenails can get more brittle.

Here is a cool post-pedicure treatment.

one-fourth a cup of water

one teaspoon of baking soda

one tablespoon of sea salt

one tablespoon of olive oil

Mix and scrub all over feet, nails and between toes after nails dry from the pedicure before wiping off.

FEET PROBLEMS CAN AFFECT YOUR WORK

I've known trainers, nurses, law enforcement officers and those in the hospitality industry who've had their careers shortened because their feet pain became unbearable.

I admit, I've neglected my feet for most of my life. I should have consulted a medical professional when I stepped on the tack when I was younger and when I suffered the stress fracture in high school that resulted in years of lingering pain. I told myself it was something that would just heal on its own. Even when I got older and experienced off and on again pain I should have sought out a podiatrist. I hated doctors and medical professionals, I had no faith in them seeing what they didn't do for my mentally ill mom when I was a kid. I also see them as authority figures and to this day I have problems with authority figures.

We do so much walking, sitting, have an abundance of salt in and sometimes having a poor overall diet - all these things causes inflammation and all this affects our feet. I've heard it a million times over the years that with my history I should take better care of my feet and by neglecting them this could be a cause of problems in my old age. Working as a sports reporter for newspapers, specifically covering college football and basketball, I did so much walking, driving, flying, walking around campuses and stadiums and arenas that it was hard on my foot at times.

Feet problems can cause lost days at work, plus produce less than productive days. A good friend worked in a spa and those long, taxing hours spent on her feet took a toll of her. As a personal fitness trainer I would sometimes have six or seven clients back-to-back and with my problematic left foot, it was tough for me at times.

And it's more than just pain you might experience at work. Continual pressure can put strains on other muscles, tendons and joints. Over time this can lead to bad posture, which I'll talk about in another chapter. The pain can cause us to walk in an unnatural way to compensate for feet discomfort, which can also cause back pain and the loss of balance.

The human foot contains twenty-six bones, thirty-three tendons and over one hundred muscles and ligaments. Common worked-related problems associated with the feet and ankles include plantar fasciitis (inflammation of the tissue running along the heel and supporting the arch), heel spurs (bony protrusions under the heel), tendinitis (pain and tenderness in the tendons), bunions (painful hard lumps), warts, corns and calluses (patches of thickened skin), flat feet, pronation and neuroma (the result of a pinched nerve between the toes).

So, what's a person to do to avoid or manage work-related feet pain?

1. Take breaks off your feet and limit long times on feet if possible.

2. Indulge yourself in self-massage or seek out professional massage treatments.

3. Consider a reflexology session, which targets specific pressure points in the feet.

4. Make sure you are wearing appropriate shoes that provide comfort and stability.

5. See a podiatrist for regular checkup and feet maintenance.

TALK TO A PODIATRIST ABOUT FEET PROBLEMS

When I went to a new podiatrist to have calluses on my feet removed and talk to him about ordering orthodic shoe inserts, I didn't want to pass up the opportunity to discuss my foot problems.

As a new patient, he was conducting a pretty detailed examination as I shared with him about the nail trauma, fungus, infections, Athlete's Feet, eczema and flat foot issues I've had that have seemed to be more exacerbated these days. He was present and engaging and told me that generally feet problems happen ten percent more often as we get older, that fungus is highly contagious and most topical creams are not successful long term.

Dr. Schmidt was his name and I could tell right away English was not his first language. He went on to tell me that while many oral medications work, many have side effects and its common to have some sort of bacterial infection when you do damage to the nail by banging it on something or repeatedly wearing ill-fitting shoes. Dr. Schmidt talked at length about treating feet and nail problems from the inside.

"I'm a big fan of supplements," said Schmidt, a cyclist and distance runner. "Whether its for the lubrication of the joints, tendons and cartilage, or just to have healthy nails growing so that we can withstand wear and tear, it helps to have a preventative attitude and look for help where you can."

Talking to him made me realize the importance of checking in with a podiatrist for routine feet care. More often if you have feet issues. He was a wealth of information and I hinged on his every word. I asked Dr. Schmidt if he knew of a simple remedy for treating nail problems and he suggested trying apple cider vinegar and vitamin E oil for both fungus and infections. He also spoke of having extra room in your shoes or if you have flat feet, are on your feet for long periods of time at work and play, and especially if you have nail damage. "When the toes and the feet are rubbing against the shoes... that is problematic," he said.

It took me years to finally see a podiatrist and I wondered if I could have saved myself some pain by going earlier in life. I remember working part-time at a speciality fitness shoe store once and a client I had as a trainer had just added running as a part of her fitness routine. She wanted me to go with her to pick out the best shoes for her and I had to force her to get larger-sized shoes to help relieve some of the pressure she had from several feet issues.

Although I didn't take my own advice, I convinced her to see a podiatrist for the various ailments she had. Eventually she was running pain free. Now I see a podiatrist at least twice a year now that I know I have arthritis-related circulation issues.

KNEE PAIN EQUALS FEET PAIN

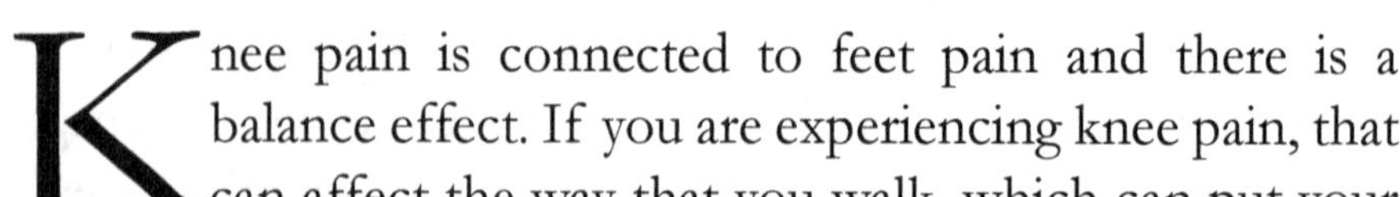

Knee pain is connected to feet pain and there is a balance effect. If you are experiencing knee pain, that can affect the way that you walk, which can put your feet, ankles and toes out of balance.

When we are younger, we have a thicker fluid protein inside our knee joints to lubricate them as we move. This fluid acts as a cushion and shock absorber inside the knee, called the synvial fluid. As we age, this fluid dries out, leaving our bones to painfully rub against and grind each other. In recent days - I'm now approaching sixty - I've experienced some discomfort in my left knee from time to time. This knee is connected to the flat foot I injured early in life. So many years of playing team sports both in high school and college, then recreationally has taken its toll on both knees really, although the left one has caused me more problems. Knee pain is the main reason I stopped running after many years.

Knee discomfort can be quite subtle at first. You might notice it when you stand from sitting, or walking up a flight of stairs, or getting in and out of a car. For me, I notice my knee pain the first thing in the morning when I get out of bed. I will say, don't be so quick to opt for surgery for that knee-related feet pain.

There are over-the-counter and prescription medications you can try, but I would say the first order of business should be exercising. There are quite a few you can start with to deal with knee-related feet pain. Studying kinesiology, the best way I can describe the connection from knee problems to feet issues is to imagine a straight line from your knees to your feet and lower back and how that line can be affected by knee pain. The body will compensate for that pain somehow. Having extra weight, being stiff and moving less, combined with a poor diet can all contribute to knee issues.

I think having one leg shorter than the other and a flat left foot eventually led to pain in my left knee as for years I was walking out of alignment. Knee problems are more common as we age and our knees are more subject to trauma as we age as well. We need to be strong and flexible in our legs, which means doing resistance training work on the glutes, quads, hamstrings and calves.

Proper footwear is key as well. When you have high arches you need more cushion in your shoes. If you have one or more flat feet like me, you need more support and rigidity in your shoes.

Some of my favorite exercises to ease knee pain includes different variations of squats and lunges, including wall squats with or without the benefit of weights, step-ups and yoga poses, especially the ones where you are standing on one leg.

THE ROLE OF EXERCISE IN SKIN AND FEET HEALTH

Exercise promotes healing, muscle tone and circulation, all great things for the skin, the largest organ in the body, including the skin on our feet. Healthy feet are nice looking. I look at exercise as medicine for the skin. The sweating that comes from exercise gets out some of the impurities in our skin, from our head down to our feet.

Feet really need resistance training like other parts of the body as resistance training can tighten the skin and cardiovascular work such as walking, running, cycling, swimming keeps the blood flowing well. Good overall circulation is tied to proper blood flow.

There are a lot of studies that talk about how exercise can slow the aging process of the signs of poor skin health. As a fitness professional, especially during the warm weather months, I've noticed seemingly healthy-looking people with unhealthy-looking feet.

Eating well and reducing the overall calorie intake are great for the skin, but in my opinion, nothing works helps like exercise. The average person's lean body mass declines with age - six percent of lean muscle is lost each decade during the adult years. That rate accelerates after age forty-five and that can show up in the skin's appearance. Fortunately, your feet don't age, in theory, like the rest of your body.

Look at it this way, our problems are going to be magnified as we age. Exercise increases metabolism, is linked to longevity, important to cellular functioning in older adults, especially immune system functioning.

The most obvious signs of aging and a lack of exercise is - wrinkled skin, age spots and dehydrated skin - these factors can really be seen on the feet. One of the reasons older people appear to have decreased weight is because of a lack of lean muscle. Again, incorporating some resistance training into the mix can go a long way in promoting overall skin health.

According to several skin care specialists I have in my reference book, there are four main causes of aged- looking skin on the feet - sun damage, smoking, having a poor overall diet and drinking too much alcohol. A lack of exercise is a close fifth.

So what if you are not really an exercise person, but want to increase metabolism and circulation in your body? How about those sluggish days when you don't feel like exercising but still want to burn some calories? A friend of mine who fancies herself as a book critic suggested I include some simple ways to burn calories doing routine stuff around the house. After initially giving her dirty looks, I decided her suggestions wasn't that bad after all.

1. Drink coffee - caffeine can help boost calorie burn for up to three hours. Perhaps try drinking it as you are sweeping or dusting.

2. Walk around your place holding a stability ball - not only good for your feet, but doing this as you move can help burn over 200 more calories daily.

3. Cut out carbohydrates twice a week from your diet - just two days of it and you'll be surprised at the calories you'll save in the long run.

4. Chew gum when you're hungry and there a chance you'll eat ten percent less.

5. Turn down the heat as the idea room temperature for melting fat is 64 degrees. This is an easy way to burn fat while you are sleeping.

6. Cook something spicy with peppers - this can spike your metabolism, which helps you burn calories.

7. Walk in place watching the news - thirty minutes goes fast and you might forget you're exercising.

8. Stay unstressed - studies indicate that stressed out people work off fewer calories that those who are calm.

9. Say no to the second glass of beer or wine - you will not only save on calories and that extra libation may slow down fat blasting.

10. Move - simply tapping your feet or pacing can move hundreds of more calories than being still.

BUILDING YOUR OWN HOME GYM

Working at various fitness stores and as an in-home personal fitness trainer, I know what it takes to build a personalized home gym. When my ex-wife, also a personal trainer, and I got married, the two of us decided we would do training in our home. We had to put our heads together to create the perfect gym for us. On a personal level I wanted to make sure I had exercises to work my lower extremities, especially my feet, as I was concerned with my posture and balance.

The fitness company I was working for at the time specialized in home gyms and individual exercise pieces that fit many different budgets. Space, interest and budget should be prime considerations when outfitting a gym. Because this is a book about feet care, I know having proper matting or flooring, one or two step-up steps, dumbbells, a simple piece of cardiovascular equipment like an exercise bike and a leg extension, a jump rope and leg press machine provide the perfect foundation for some feet-centric workout. Overall, there are many decisions that need to be made to ensure you have the perfect home fitness environment. It's easier to train your feet the more options you have.

The following are some considerations for building your own individualized home gym.

1. Put your exercise stuff in the biggest room of your place that you feel comfortable in. You need room to jump around and move freely and a room that has ventilation and a small room can cramp your enthusiasm and motivation.

2. Invest in a full-length mirror. Not for vanity sake, but to make sure you can watch yourself and make sure you are doing your exercises right and you have good form. This is particularly important when you are doing exercises that affect the feet like squats, lunges and balance-related moves like standing on one leg.

3. Have some of sound system for listening to music, or in my case, talk radio, to distract you, especially if you are doing cardiovascular work.

4. Have your home gym area brightly painted with good lighting to help provide positive energy.

5. When it comes to cardiovascular equipment, if you are to have one piece of equipment, make sure you select something that will challenge you, whether it's a bike, elliptical or treadmill.

6. Invest in some inexpensive essentials that promote variety, such as a jump rope, exercise bands, dumbbells and a medicine ball, for example. All are really good for legs, ankles and feet exercises. Go to a store that specializes in fitness equipment to get the best stuff and a warranty. Kettle bells, a

ViPR and BOSU balls have become popular these days with more advanced folks or those looking for more of a challenge.

7. Be sure to have the basics - weights, a mat, a bench and/or a stability ball. Have enough stuff to work your body from head to toe.

Again, shop around, but don't cheap out because not all quality is the same at the stores. You size should be a factor in picking machines. Those on a budget can still outfit a functional gym.

Nutrition for the skin in general

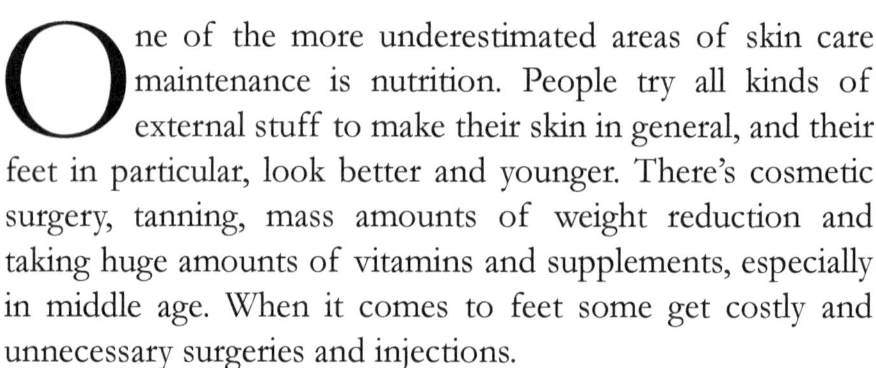

One of the more underestimated areas of skin care maintenance is nutrition. People try all kinds of external stuff to make their skin in general, and their feet in particular, look better and younger. There's cosmetic surgery, tanning, mass amounts of weight reduction and taking huge amounts of vitamins and supplements, especially in middle age. When it comes to feet some get costly and unnecessary surgeries and injections.

I'm a big fan of vitamins and supplements as I know you don't always have the time to eat right even if you strive to live a fit life. Nutrition for the skin and particularly the feet is even more important if you are diabetic or overweight. Diabetics are prone to dry skin because of dehydration and other factors. Extra weight puts pressure on certain parts of the feet, allowing the skin in those areas to get damaged.

Nutrition for the skin starts with making sure you are properly hydrated. Strive to drink at least half of your bodyweight in ounces of water daily, and that is a minimal requirement. Tea and coffee is OK, but water is best. Incorporate more water-based foods in your diet like melons and cucumbers. Liquids with lots of sugar and salt can dry out skin and cause inflammation. Same goes for alcoholic beverages.

You need a variety-filled diet full of fruits and vegetables. The more colors in your food the better.

Many people have argued with me that nutrition doesn't play much of a role in feet health. I would often refer clients and others I got tired of arguing with to Dana, a personal trainer friend of mine who is also a clinical nutritionist. She was my running buddy when we both worked at a hospital-based fitness center who was instrumental in talking me into running in my first half-marathon.

Dana used to be skinny fat until she tweaked her diet. It wasn't that she ate badly, just not enough of the right stuff. She used to have pain in her knees, calves and feet and got cramps often.

"I should have known better I was getting too much salt, not enough potassium, not enough fruits and I had a lot of inflammation in my lower half of my body," she said. " I had so many aches and pains in my feet and that went slowly away when I started making sounder nutritional choices."

Like me, Dana was also a fan of having super foods in her diet - fish, berries, leafy greens, fish, beans and grains - which she said are intended to decrease inflammation, promote healing and helps with digestion.

"A lot of those aches and pains in the feet can come from being undernourished and lacking in vitamins and minerals,"

Dana said. "Which also adds to poor circulation and retaining water, so the feet swell and cause other issues in your shoes."

Your source of your foods is going to be your fuel, so it's really important for your energy, strength, stamina and recovery, so be smart what you put in your body.

As a trainer, I've seen and heard people complain about the swelling they get in their feet. I tell them it's mostly because of inflammation from the foods they eat.

How we eat has so much to do with feet care. That inflammation that ignites other issues in the feet often gets ignored. Something simple like carrying too much weight can cause inflammatory actions in the feet that can result in making simple things like just walking uncomfortable.

Often we reach for what's available and consume too much fast, prepacked and processed food loaded with sugar, fat, salt and too many calories.

When it comes to feet care and your diet, consider meal prepping too, getting rid of trigger foods in the house and consuming lots of lean meats, green vegetables, fruits and healthy grains. Making sure you get enough protein to have strong muscles in the legs, calves and feet.

Joint pain, arthritis and obesity are closely related to inflammation. Foods that contribute to inflammation in the feet include trans fats and processed meats. I can remember the swelling, dehydration, aches and pains in my feet and the rest of my body when I ate crappy for an extended period of time.

Here are a list of some power foods to have in your diet that provide good nutrition to the skin and feet.:

Acai berries, apples, nuts, asparagus, avocado, berries, cherries, cinnamon, cauliflower, cranberries, citrus fruits, fish, edaname, oatmeal, tomatoes, peppers, eggs, watermelon and brown rice.

These are foods high in water content, have antioxidants, fiber, protein, potassium, vitamins and minerals and many are antifungal, antibacterial and provide healthy Omega-3 fatty acids to promote circulation.

I also want to say something about collagen. Healthy servings of foods packed with proteins, vitamins and minerals can amp up your body's supply of collagen, the most plentiful protein in the body. It's in your muscles, bones, tendons, ligaments and other connective tissues, so you can see how important it is to feet maintenance.

Collagen levels decrease as you get older, contributing to stiffer, less flexible tendons and ligaments, shrinking, weakening muscles, joint pain or osteoarthritis due to worn cartilage.

Weak leg muscles can lead to weak knees, ankles and feet.

It's important to consume protein-rich foods. When your body makes collagen, it combines amino acids - nutrients you get from eating protein-rich foods. Foods packed full of proteins include: beef, chicken, fish, beans, eggs and dairy products.

Making collagen also requires vitamin C, which you can get by eating citrus fruits, red and green peppers, tomatoes and dark and leafy greens. Your body also needs zinc and copper and these minerals can be found in meats, shellfish, nuts, whole grains and beans.

FOODS TO HELP BLOATING FEET

People have asked me often how to get rid of the bloat they've experienced in their feet, especially at times when they've consider themselves healthy eaters. As I mentioned earlier, certain healthy foods can cause gas and water retention and that can especially be an issue for your feet. I can think of times I experienced bloating in my lower extremities in general, and my feet in particular, while at work, running, cycling, playing basketball or simply walking and how uncomfortable it was.

When you are bloated you feel heavy and look bigger than you actually are. I asked around and tried a lot of foods in experimentation and I have complied what I think are ten foods that can help you beat the bloat. The main thing here is you want foods to keep things moving through your digestive system.

1. **Grapefruit** - It helps to pull in carbohydrates for they can be used as fuel.

2. **Lemons** - Try adding some in your water, they help speed up metabolism.

3. **Watermelon** - A natural water reducer that's loaded with vitamins.

4. **Peppers -** The hotter the better. They also help speed up metabolism.

5. **Avocados** - They have healthy fat to absorb and move foods around.

6. **Olive oil** - Another healthy fat to have in the body.

7. **Almonds** - High in fiber and protein and helps speed food through the body.

8. **Flax seeds** - Also high in fiber and healthy fats.

9, **Cinnamon** - Helps regulate blood sugar levels and a natural blood thinner.

10. **Vinegar** - Good for the skin and helps break down food.

All of these foods are regular staples in my diet and do help reduce bloating in my body and feet, when I consume them consistently. Grapefruit, lemons and watermelon are especially helpful because they are high water content foods, which helps to regulate weight and keep food passing through the body. Other bloat killers are fruit and vegetable smoothies, green tea and probiotic foods like sauerkraut and kimchi and Kefir, a fermented dairy beverage that I love to make smoothies with.

It helps to eat for satiety, stuff like fruits, vegetables, whole grains, lean proteins, beans, nuts and seeds, and avoid sugar, fat and salt, which leads to bloat.

Bloat can also come from stress, medications and too much alcohol.

SARCOPENIA AND THE EFFECTS ON THE FEET

I'll try not to get overly complicated talking about sarcopenia, which is basically age-related muscle loss. I had never heard of this word until I started working on my senior fitness certification.

As I've gotten older, I find it harder to maintain muscle tone and mass despite making a concentrated effort. There were times I ignored the pain I got from going at weight training so hard, remembering the days when I had the bodyfat of a greyhound. I watch my cardiovascular training and monitor my diet, but unfortunately starting around age 35 we begin losing one percent of our muscle mass every year. This stinks because as we age we are more prone to injury as our ligaments and tendons stiffens and cartilage thins. We also have a decline in reaction time and bone density.

Our bodies are master compensators and it doesn't take much for a person to start reversing the effects of sarcopenia, which results in the loss of strength. Sarcopenia puts older persons at risk of sustaining agalls or simply being unable to care for themselves.

Sarcopenia as it relates to the feet can not only result in pains and possible injuries, but balance issues and problems walking and standing.

Keeping stress out of your body is a good start at battling this. Watch out for anxiety and depression as poor mental health management goes a long way in your body's functioning and level of inflammation. I saw stress and depression in clients starting in their early 40s working as a personal fitness trainer at several hospital-based fitness centers. Many of them were middle age or older and not only fighting depression but the fact they were losing muscle at an alarming rate.

I've seen clients with unstable balance, weak legs, ankles calves and feet from inactivity, injuries and poor circulation.

Next you need to eat mindfully, getting enough protein, fiber and water in your diet. Your lower extremities, including your feet, have muscles that lose strength, mass and flexibility. Not all calories are created equally, same with hydration. You need carbohydrates for fuel and then again, not all of them are created equally as well.

You should engage in some kind of resistance and stretching training and that could be yoga, bodyweight exercises, using weights or bands. Since I'm taking about feet here, a loss of strength in your feet can lead to many concerns. Your feet health connects to your posture and balance. It connects to the core too. Bad back and feet can make you miserable. I encouraged folks to work their entire posterior chain - that's the group of muscles connected to the lower back, glutes, hamstrings, calves and quadriceps.

Core exercises include standing and seated twists, side bends, knee lifts and crunches. Lower body exercises can include leg extensions, leg presses, heel raises, calf raises, variations of squats, ankle rotations and flexion movements, standing and holding on balls of feet and flexing the toes.

There is a chain reaction from the core, legs and feet as it relates to sarcopenia. Some possible negative effects include uneven wear of shoes, arthritis, corns, bunions, hammer toes, sprained ankles, heel spurs, plantar faciitis and general feet pain.